P9-EMG-449

Heart Smart

a plan for low-cholesterol living

About the Author

GAIL BECKER, a registered dietitian, earned her degree in dietetics from Drexel University. She has managed the food and nutrition department of the world's largest weight-control organization, directed dietetics at a large metropolitan hospital, and headed dietetic services for a major food company.

Ms. Becker currently serves on the Subcommittee on Nutrition Program of the American Heart Association and is a member of the American Dietetic Association, the Society for Nutrition Education, American College of Nutrition, the Institute of Food Technology, the American Home Economics Association, and many other professional organizations. She conducts nutrition seminars and appears frequently on television and radio programs as an authority on nutrition. Her published articles have appeared in leading women's magazines.

Ms. Becker is the president of a Great Neck, New York–based public relations/marketing communications company serving the food and nutrition industry.

Heart Smart

a plan for low-cholesterol living

by Gail L. Becker, R.D.

Introduction by
Scott Grundy, M.D., Ph.D.

supported by
Merrell Dow
Merrell Dow Pharmaceuticals Inc.

PUBLISHED BY POCKET BOOKS NEW YORK

Another *Original* publication of POCKET BOOKS

POCKET BOOKS, a division of Simon & Schuster, Inc.
1230 Avenue of the Americas, New York, N.Y. 10020

Copyright © 1984 by Merrell Dow Pharmaceuticals, Inc.

. All rights reserved, including the right to reproduce
this book or portions thereof in any form whatsoever.
For information address Pocket Books, 1230 Avenue
of the Americas, New York, N.Y. 10020

ISBN: 0-671-30924-2

Second Pocket Books Special Printing August, 1984

10 9 8 7 6 5 4 3 2

POCKET and colophon are registered trademarks
of Simon & Schuster, Inc.

Printed in the U.S.A.

Acknowledgments

I would like to thank Scott M. Grundy, M.D., Ph.D., from the University of Texas Health Science Center, and John Foreyt, Ph.D., from the Baylor College of Medicine, for their contribution to the preparation of this book.

My thanks also to Laura W. Conway, M.S., and Marsha Hudnall, M.S., R.D., for their invaluable assistance and endless hours of dedication in helping me put it all together.

Acknowledgments would not be complete without reference to Merrell Dow Pharmaceuticals Inc., whose commitment to cardiovascular health made this book possible.

CONTENTS

* * *

Tables

Introduction

by Scott M. Grundy, M.D., Ph.D.

Scott M. Grundy, M.D., Ph.D., is Professor of Internal Medicine and Biochemistry and Director of the Center for Human Nutrition at the University of Texas Health Science Center. Dr. Grundy is also Immediate Past Chairman and member of the Nutrition Committee of the American Heart Association.

"It's just aging. Nothing much you can do about that."

"My parents were both overweight. No sense trying to fight it."

"Exercise? I tried jogging, but it hurt my knees."

These statements are from people who have been diagnosed as having atherosclerosis, a disease in which blood vessels are narrowed or occluded by deposits of cholesterol. However factual they may be, their statements may be no more than excuses for not taking control of their lives and doing something about their condition.

If you have atherosclerosis, now is the time to make the most important decision of your life, for your life. That decision is to accept the things you cannot change—factors such as heredity and aging that may or may not have contributed to your disease—and decide to change whatever factors you can for the possibility of a healthier future.

If your car doesn't work, you usually do something about it. For example, when particles in the car's fuel line block the flow of gasoline to the engine, you probably take it to the service station to be repaired.

In atherosclerosis, fatty deposits are cutting down the flow of blood to your heart and other parts of your body, which cannot function properly without sufficient blood supply. When you think of your body as being more important than your car, your choice is clear. You must work to change factors adversely influencing your health. This means replacing less than good habits that contribute to your condition with good ones, and it takes time and effort.

There's little you can do about natural aging. And you can't pick your parents. But you can stop smoking. You can lose weight. You may improve your heart's efficiency. You may lower the amount of cholesterol in your blood. You can take control of your behavior patterns and make a choice for a healthier life—and a longer one.

In atherosclerosis, fatty deposits form on the arterial wall, causing narrowing of the passageway and retardation of blood flow. Once cholesterol deposition begins, the artery is injured, and scarring can occur, enlarging the obstruction. Cholesterol makes up the major portion of this deposition or plaque, along with smaller amounts of triglycerides. Table A depicts the stages of atherosclerosis.

TABLE A
Stages of Atherosclerosis

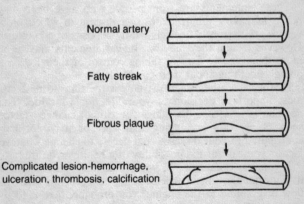

Normal artery

Fatty streak

Fibrous plaque

Complicated lesion-hemorrhage, ulceration, thrombosis, calcification

SOURCE Grundy, Scott M., M.D.; "Atherosclerosis: Pathology, Pathogenesis, and Role of Risk Factors." *Disease-A-Month*, Year Book Medical Publishers, Inc., Chicago, Illinois, 1983.

Although cholesterol is required for the normal function of cell membranes, high blood cholesterol causes the disease to progress faster, increasing chances of a heart attack or stroke. For this reason, high blood cholesterol is considered a major risk factor for coronary heart disease and stroke. Since large amounts of triglycerides are not found in the atherosclerotic plaque, high triglycerides are a questionable risk factor. Epidemiological studies have, in general, failed to identify elevated triglycerides as a primary, significant, independent risk factor for coronary heart disease.

Your physician determines whether or not your blood cholesterol is too high by measuring your level of blood cholesterol and then comparing it to guidelines. The American Medical Association Council on Scientific Affairs recently recommended that people with blood cholesterol levels in the top half (50th percentile) of the population could benefit from cholesterol reduction and that people whose levels are in the top tenth (90th percentile) of the population deserve vigorous dietary therapy and, most likely, concurrent drug treatment. Table B shows those levels as they vary by age and sex.

TABLE B
MEDIAN CHOLESTEROL LEVELS

| | Men | | Women | |
| | Cholesterol Level (mg/dl) | | Cholesterol Level (mg/dl) | |
Age	50th	90th	50th	90th
20–29	172	215	164	207
30–39	194	234	176	219
40–49	206	254	195	241
50–59	211	261	222	275
60–69	210	258	228	280
70–79	205	249	228	280

Source: Lipid Research Clinics data, *Journal of the American Medical Association* 250:14, October 14, 1983.

Various fatty substances in the body can contribute to a higher cholesterol level. In addition, some fats that you eat seem to actually cause increased cholesterol levels. The most common are saturated fats, which are found in animal sources such as meat, eggs, butter, and other dairy products. Some plant sources, such as coconut and palm oils and cocoa butter, are also rich in saturated fats.

Other fats seem to lower blood cholesterol. Polyunsaturated fats, such as corn oil and safflower oil, come mainly from plant sources. When polyunsaturated fats are taken in place of saturated fats, the plasma cholesterol is lowered.

Recent studies show another kind of fat, called monounsaturated fat, also lowers cholesterol levels. One major source of this fat is olive oil.

So you can see that making changes in your diet—a factor that's completely under your control—can lower the cholesterol in your body.

Other major risk factors are:

- Cigarette smoking
- Obesity
- Lack of exercise
- High blood pressure
- Diabetes mellitus

In anyone with a high cholesterol level, these additional risk factors can be extremely dangerous, and all of the five can be controlled. And you're the one who can do it.

Smoking is an extremely important risk factor and, like diet, one that can be controlled by the patient. One theory of the way smoking increases risk is that it damages the arterial wall and allows more cholesterol from the bloodstream to enter the artery. Another theory is that smoking leads to the formation of blood clots in partially obstructed coronary arteries.

Obesity contributes still another hazard. It probably acts to produce abnormal fats in the bloodstream, which cause changes leading to atherosclerosis.

Lack of exercise, via obesity, may also escalate your chances of developing heart disease. Traditionally, studies have shown that exercise itself is a protective factor against heart disease.

High blood pressure is another major risk factor and, again, one that can be controlled. Even mild elevations of blood pressure can double the risk of heart attack. High blood pressure seems to force cholesterol into the arterial wall and promote its deposition. Another way in which high blood pressure may cause atherosclerosis and subsequent coronary heart disease is by damaging the artery, allowing for increased deposits of cholesterol.

Diabetes, another significant element in the picture, may cause damage that increases the chances of heart attack and decreased blood flow to the extremities.

All these are dangerous in anyone who has high levels of cholesterol. Risk factors are multiplicative: the more you have, the greater your chances of developing atherosclerosis. The risk factors act in different ways, but the end result is the same. Table C graphically illustrates the predicted incidence of heart disease occurrence.

TABLE C
Heart Disease Combined Risk Factors

The Danger of Heart Attack and Stroke Increases with
the Number of Risk Factors Present
(Example 45 year old male)

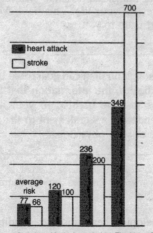

SOURCE: American Heart Association, *The Heart Book*.
American Heart Association, Dallas, 1980.

Changing your diet is a vital step toward better health. Take charge today, keeping these goals in mind:

- Achieve or maintain ideal body weight
- Decrease total fat intake
- Reduce saturated fat and cholesterol intake
- Decrease sodium consumption

In addition to a controlled diet, a physician may decide that a patient requires drug therapy, specifically designed to lower cholesterol. Drug therapy is especially indicated when diet alone does not reduce the cholesterol level to an acceptable range, as indicated on page 11.

Your doctor has made the diagnosis of elevated blood cholesterol. Now he or she can help you by advising you on diet and monitoring your progress. In some cases, the physician will rely on the help of a registered dietitian. But it is up to you to effect the changes necessary for your own better health. Only you can make the conscious decision to adhere to a diet program. Your physician may recommend a combination of diet and drugs to help you reach and maintain a desired serum cholesterol level. In that case, it's also up to you to follow your doctor's directions and together find the treatment program that works best for you.

You can make things happen that will lead to improved health for the rest of your life. This book will help you get started. The rest is up to you.

> **Although no plan can guarantee better health, the information that follows may be of help to you. It is intended as a supplement to the advice of your physician.**

Heart Smart

a plan for low-cholesterol living

CHAPTER I

EATING FOR HEART HEALTH

As you start on your plan to change habits acquired over a lifetime, it's encouraging to realize you have plenty of company.

Since the early 1960s, millions of Americans have learned about the risks of atherosclerosis and coronary heart disease, and have successfully changed their lifestyles.

The American Heart Association reports that since 1964 the average per capita intake of saturated fat and cholesterol has declined and, correspondingly, cholesterol levels in adults have decreased. Millions of American adults have stopped smoking. Of the estimated 34 million American adults with high blood pressure, the proportion of the population who actively control this risk factor has risen from 10 percent to 50 percent or higher.[1]

As mentioned in the Introduction, cholesterol is necessary to a healthy body. It acts as an insulator of nerve and brain tissue. An important part of the cell membrane, it makes your skin almost completely waterproof, while at the same time retarding evaporation of water from the body.

Since your body needs cholesterol, it ensures a supply by manufacturing it. But when a high dietary intake of cholesterol is added to your body's naturally produced cholesterol, your system may become overloaded.

Diet is the major key to reducing cholesterol and controlling atherosclerosis. A regular weight-control program, integrating diet and exercise, takes commitment. As you progressively change your habits, making your plan part of a permanent lifestyle, it becomes easier and easier until it is second nature.

The importance of diet in lowering body cholesterol can be seen in recent studies. A group of researchers at the University of Minnesota has found that vegetarian diets containing no animal fats result in lower blood cholesterol levels.[2]

In studies of Japan's population, it seems that increasing Westernization in that nation has been accompanied by an increase in death from heart disease. Compared to the U.S. population, Japanese in Japan have low cholesterol levels. However, Japanese living in California and eating American diets have relatively high cholesterol levels, and the severity of atherosclerosis approaches that of Caucasians in the United States.[3]

Other studies performed around the world confirm that blood cholesterol levels are elevated by dietary cholesterol and saturated fat, and that certain changes in dietary habits can lower blood cholesterol and the risk of heart disease—this nation's number one killer today.

The good news is that Americans are becoming more aware of the relationship between diet and disease. In fact, the most sweeping change Americans have made in their lifestyle over the past ten years has concerned food habits.[4]

As a nation, we are eating more vegetables, fruit, fish, and chicken, and fewer animal fats such as beef, butter, and dairy products. The latter foods have been status symbols in the affluent industrial countries, which have traditionally had the highest incidence of heart disease.[5,6,7]

Between 1963 and 1977, per capita consumption of animal fats fell almost 50 percent in America. Perhaps this accounts for the dramatic drop in heart disease among adult Americans.[8]

Modifying your eating and other lifestyle habits is discussed in Chapters II and IV. It is up to you and your doctor to determine the combination of diet and exercise that fits into your future life/health plan. In the meantime, such changes for the general public are a topic of debate among scientists.

Some researchers believe that there should be major changes across the board in the American diet. Others think it would be premature to recommend any changes at all. A more moderate approach is taken by those who advocate individual prescription. These health professionals have concluded that evidence suggests a relationship between diet and coronary heart disease. But they agree that the risks don't apply to everyone.

Individual prescription—a diet combined with an exercise program and possible drug therapy based on a physician's judgment as to the special health needs of each patient—seems to be the most sensible approach.

We all know persons who have changed their lives through diet and exercise, and have adopted a missionary zeal toward converting friends who haven't yet "seen the light." The truth is, not everyone needs to change.

You, on the other hand, have been told by your doctor that you have a cholesterol level which is too high. So you know the time has come to make a choice. The most exciting aspect of choosing a healthier approach is that you, yourself, can make it happen.

CHAPTER II

CHANGING LIFESTYLES: EATING AND EXERCISING

by John Foreyt, Ph.D.

Dr. John Foreyt is Director of the Diet Modification Clinic at the Baylor College of Medicine, Houston, Texas.

Changing a diet that you have been eating for years isn't always as simple as it may sound. Ingrained eating habits influence just what and how much you eat to a great degree.

The first step in putting a new diet plan into action is to take a look at your eating habits. Also consider why you've developed these habits. The key to success is replacing negative habits with positive behavior.

The main reason so many diet and exercise weight-control programs fail is that people often think of them as a temporary inconvenience, a necessary evil designed to take off weight by the wedding, before summer, by the holidays. When the diet is over, it's back to the same old eating patterns that caused all the trouble in the first place.

Doctors agree that the only way to take weight off and keep it off is to make basic lifestyle changes. At the Diet Modification Clinic at the Baylor College of Medicine in Houston, Texas, we teach patients to do this through a process called behavior modification—changing your behavior patterns and long-standing eating habits.

We have devised a plan to teach people how to take control of their eating habits. After two months of behavior modification sessions aimed at changing eating behavior, about three-quarters of the overweight patients were able to maintain their weight loss or continue to lose. Our studies have followed these patients up to a year. In this chapter, we will share with you many of the tips included in the Baylor program, to aid you in making positive changes in your behavior.

How to Begin

With your doctor, select a good diet—one low in cholesterol, saturated fat, and sodium, like the Heart Smart Diet outlined in Chapter III. Then begin your behavior modification program as outlined below, so that you can incorporate your diet plan into your life plan.

The Dietary Detective

To change your eating habits, you must first identify them. Each day write everything you eat and drink in a small notebook, or photocopy the Food Record Sheet at the end of this chapter (Table IIC) and use it to keep a complete record of everything that goes into your mouth. This means not just at mealtime, but all the time. Don't forget that bite of tuna you took while you were making sandwiches. Or the tasting you did to make sure the stew was seasoned just right. Or the three crackers you grabbed after you came in the door tonight just to "tide you over" until dinner. Note the time of day you had the food, where you ate, your mood when you ate each item, and with whom you ate. If you are dieting to lose pounds, keep a record of your weight. Hang a sheet of graph paper near the scale, and weigh yourself each day at the same time, noting your own ups and downs (see sample in Table IIA). The numbers on the vertical axis should range from your present weight to your goal weight in intervals of one to five pounds.

After two weeks, study your food records to see which habits can coexist with your new diet and which need changing. Look for patterns. Find foods not permitted on your low-cholesterol, low-saturated fat, reduced-sodium eating plan.

Once you've identified self-defeating habits that have become part of your behavior, you're well on the way to changing those habits.

Deliberate Detours and Pink Pigs

Your next step is to find ways to change your environment. If you regularly stop at a neighborhood deli on your way to work to pick up a Danish and coffee, take a different route to the office and thus avoid the impulse to stop. Don't keep off-limits snacks in the house. If another family member wants them, he or she will have to get them somewhere else.

Put notes to yourself on the mirror or refrigerator with the notation: "Those who indulge bulge." I have one patient who has decorated her refrigerator door with pink pig magnets that say, "You back again?" and "I'm getting thin s l o w l y."

Choose one place to eat when you're at home and eat every meal there. Devote your entire attention to eating. This means no phone calls, television, letter writing, or reading. *Never* eat standing up. Eliminate food cues by removing anything from your environment that causes you to eat what you shouldn't. Some examples are television commercials that present an opportunity to get a snack, office birthday cakes, certain times of day that signal snack time, and other persons eating near you.

The Strategic Planner

Use various strategies to control your eating habits. One of these might be writing a contract with yourself. If you lose two pounds this week, you'll treat yourself to that movie you've been wanting to see. Or buy a new shirt. Or have your hair done. You can also make a pact with your spouse or a friend. One woman's husband promised to take her on a world cruise if she'd lose thirty pounds. She did, and they went. Most of us can't afford round-the-world trips, but we can afford breakfast in bed, new clothes, books, or records. Make it fun—something nice you can anticipate.

Another effective strategy can take the form of stress reduction. In recording your moods, you may find that you're experiencing stress, boredom, loneliness, hostility, or other negative emotions in conjunction with food binges.

22

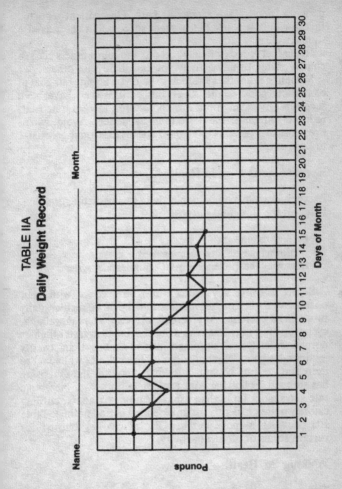

TABLE IIA
Daily Weight Record

Name _____   Month _____

Pounds

Days of Month

To ease stress, use a relaxation technique. Sit back, close your eyes, and focus on a pleasant scene, excluding anything else from your thoughts. Stay this way for five minutes. Whenever you feel stressed, take a personal time-out. Go someplace quiet, whether it's your bedroom or the lounge at work, and use this technique.

When you have negative feelings that are leading you to eat, substitute another pleasurable activity for eating. Telephone a friend. Take a relaxing bath. One patient reported that not only was her diet a great success, but she was also squeaky clean.

If you feel bored or lonely, get out and join a fitness class, a church group, or any activity you can share with others.

Modeling is another strategy to help you attain your goal of continuing good health. Seek out persons who have been successful in staying on a low-cholesterol, low-saturated fat, reduced-sodium diet and use them as models. Avoid, whenever possible, persons to whom a social occasion is an excuse to "pig out."

Exercise Your Way to Health

Exercise is a vital companion activity to any dieting program. It serves the threefold purpose of:

- Burning calories
- Improving muscle tone (fighting flab)
- Improving the efficiency of your cardiovascular system

Before starting any exercise program, check with your doctor. With his or her permission, begin a regular daily program of exercise. Any aerobic exercise, such as walking, cycling, or jogging, that causes the heart to beat faster than its normal rate for a sustained period—more than twenty minutes—is good. Not only does it burn calories while you're exercising, but its benefits last for hours after the exercising has stopped. Following your exercise period, your metabolic rate stays more rapid than usual for up to six hours, burning calories more efficiently for an extended period of time. Table IIB provides a more detailed list of calories burned for various forms of physical activity.

Walking for Health

The most accessible, easiest, and least expensive means of aerobic exercise is fast walking. Walking is also easy on the body, avoiding the shock to the bones and joints experienced in activities like jogging. And walking can be done just outside your home, without any special equipment or clothing. Walking at a good clip can burn about six calories a minute.

ENERGY EXPENDITURE CHART

Activity	Approximate Number of Calories Used Per Hour
Lying down or sleeping	80
Sitting	100
Driving a car	120
Standing	140
Domestic work	180
Walking, 2½ mph	210
Bicycling, 5½ mph	210
Gardening	220
Golf, mowing the lawn	250
Bowling	270
Walking, 3¾ mph	300
Swimming, ½ mph	300
Square dancing, volleyball, roller skating	350
Wood chopping	400
Tennis	420
Skiing, 10 mph	600
Squash or handball	600
Bicycling, 13 mph	660
Running, 10 mph	900

Source: Figures are for a 150-pound person and are based on material prepared by Robert E. Johnson, M.D., Ph.D., and colleagues, University of Illinois.

After a checkup by your doctor, start walking briskly about 15 minutes a day, three days a week. Gradually build this up to 45 minutes a day, three or four days a week. If you set aside a specific time each day, you'll be forming another good habit on the road to improved health and fitness.

Success in the Long Run

As you follow your diet and exercise plan, eating should be less important to you as a source of pleasure and satisfaction. For those times when you may overindulge during holidays and on vacations, lose weight before, not afterwards. The old excuse about eating today and dieting tomorrow is a delusion. Believe it and you will be fighting excess weight again.

If you have dropped several pounds, don't keep those baggy clothes around. Indulge in a little vanity. Buy some flattering new outfits for the slimmer you. Participate in activities you've always thought you would like: bowl, swim, exercise, cycle. Try new hobbies and activities. Enjoy the variety your new lifestyle has opened up for you.

TABLE IIC
FOOD RECORD

Name _____
Date _____

Time/Place	Emotion/With Whom	Food, Preparation and Amount	Food Group

CHAPTER III

THE HEART SMART PLAN

Now that you know how to modify your eating habits and other lifestyle behaviors in order to better your health, let's talk about a special diet which can help reduce the risk of heart disease.

Too few people realize or consider that the food we eat today affects our health in both the long and the short run, today and tomorrow. As you have already learned, many of the components of foods have an impact upon the development of atherosclerosis, the precursor of coronary heart or artery disease. Too much cholesterol, saturated fat, and sodium in our diets can increase our chances of developing heart disease. Additionally, if obesity occurs in conjunction with high cholesterol levels, high saturated fat levels, smoking, or hypertension, coronary heart disease risk is significantly increased. Table IIIA graphically compares the percentages of cholesterol and fat in the typical American diet versus that in the Heart Smart Plan.

A diet that controls the amount of fat, cholesterol, sodium, and calories can help reduce the risk of developing coronary heart disease. In order to reduce the amount of saturated fat and cholesterol in your diet, decrease the amount of animal products you eat, such as eggs, whole milk, cheese, beef, pork, and organ meats, as well as fats and oils. Such changes will also help control calories. However, if you do not need to

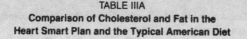

TABLE IIIA
Comparison of Cholesterol and Fat in the Heart Smart Plan and the Typical American Diet

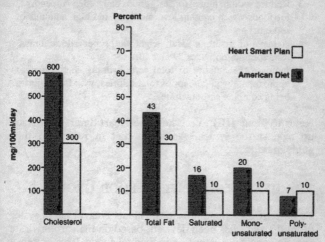

SOURCE *Dietary Goals for the United States*, prepared by the U.S. Senate Select Committee on Nutrition and Human Needs, 1977.

lose weight, you should increase your intake of complex carbohydrates, such as vegetables, fruits, grains, and legumes to make up for significant decreases in calories.

Oftentimes, a reduced sodium intake necessitates an increased potassium intake. Potassium, however, is widely distributed in many foods, particularly vegetables, fruits, dried beans, dried peas, lentils, and nuts. Getting enough potassium should not be a problem as long as you eat a well-balanced, varied diet, such as the one recommended in the Healthy Heart Plan.

The Heart Smart Plan is based on the following guidelines for helping to reduce the risk of heart disease.[9]

1. Reduce total fat calories to approximately 30 percent, with less than 10 percent from saturated fats, up to 10 percent from polyunsaturated fats, and the remainder from mono-unsaturated fats. (See Appendix B for the types of fats in fat products.)
2. Reduce cholesterol intake to less than 300 milligrams per day.

(See Appendix A for foods which contain low, medium, and high amounts of cholesterol.)

3. Reduce sodium intake to 2 to 3 grams daily. (See Appendix C for foods which contain low, medium, and high amounts of sodium.)

4. Achieve or maintain ideal weight via proper caloric intake. (See formula on pages 39 and 40.)

5. Increase the amount of total carbohydrates in the diet to approximately 55 percent of total calories, with the majority being complex carbohydrates.

Refer to Table IIIB to see how the Heart Smart Plan stacks up against the typical American diet in regard to these guidelines.

THE HEART SMART PLAN FOOD GROUPS

To simplify choosing foods in the Heart Smart Plan, a system of food groups has been devised, based on the carbohydrate, protein, and fat content of individual foods. This system is devised by nutritionists to ensure a properly balanced diet. First familiarize yourself with the groups, then use the suggested plans on pages 44–46.

VEGETABLES

As excellent sources of vitamins, minerals, complex carbohydrates, and fiber, vegetables are vital to heart health. To get the most from vegetables nutritionally, eat them raw or minimally cooked (steamed). Keep in mind that each vegetable provides different vitamins and minerals, making variety important. As a rule, if the outer portion of the vegetable is edible, that's where you'll find the majority of vitamins and minerals.

One unit in the vegetable group equals ½ cup cooked or 1 medium vegetable. Choices include:

artichoke
asparagus**
bamboo shoots
beets

TABLE IIIB
Percent of Calories from Nutrients

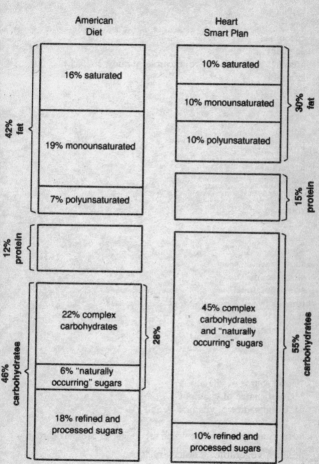

American Diet

- 42% fat
  - 16% saturated
  - 19% monounsaturated
  - 7% polyunsaturated
- 12% protein
- 46% carbohydrates
  - 28%
    - 22% complex carbohydrates
    - 6% "naturally occurring" sugars
  - 18% refined and processed sugars

Heart Smart Plan

- 30% fat
  - 10% saturated
  - 10% monounsaturated
  - 10% polyunsaturated
- 15% protein
- 55% carbohydrates
  - 45% complex carbohydrates and "naturally occurring" sugars
  - 10% refined and processed sugars

SOURCE: *Dietary Goals for the United States*, prepared by the U.S. Senate Select Committee on Nutrition and Human Needs, 1977.

broccoli***
Brussels sprouts
cabbage**
carrot*
cauliflower
celery
cucumber
eggplant
greens***(collard, endive, escarole, lettuce, spinach)
kohlrabi
leeks
mushrooms
okra
onion
parsnip
peas
peppers***
pumpkin*
radish
rutabaga
scallions
shallots
squash*
snow peas
string beans
sweet potatoes*
tomato**
turnips**
water chestnuts
yams*
zucchini

*Good source of vitamin A
**Good source of vitamin C
***Good source of vitamins A and C

NOTE: Starchy vegetables which are higher in complex carbohydrates are found in the grains group.

FRUITS

As with vegetables, some fruits are good sources of many nutrients, including carbohydrates and fiber. In addition, fruits, unlike most desserts, can satisfy your sweet tooth without tipping the scales. Also unlike many desserts, fruits provide our bodies with a variety of important vitamins and minerals. Right column indicates unit amount for each. Choices include:

apple, fresh	1 small
juice	⅓ cup
sauce	½ cup
apricots,* fresh	2 medium
canned in own juice	2 medium
dried	4 halves
banana	½ small
berries,** except strawberries	½ cup
strawberries	¾ cup
cherries	10 large
dates	2
figs, fresh and dried	2 large
fruit cocktail, fresh or canned	½ cup
grapefruit,** fresh	½ small
canned in own juice	½ cup
juice	½ cup
grapes	15 medium
kiwi**	1 medium
kumquats	4 medium
mango	½ small
melon,*** except watermelon	½ cup
watermelon	1 cup
nectarine***	1 medium
orange,** fresh	1 small
Mandarin sections	½ cup
juice	½ cup
papaya	½ cup
peach,* fresh	1 medium
canned in own juice	½ cup
pear, fresh	1 small
canned in own juice	½ cup
persimmon	1 medium
pineapple, fresh	2 slices or ½ cup
canned in own juice	2 slices or ½ cup
juice	½ cup
plums	2 medium
prunes	2 medium

raisins	2 tablespoons
tangerine**	1 large

*Good source of vitamin A
**Good source of vitamin C
***Good source of vitamins A and C

GRAINS

Foods in this group are excellent sources of complex carbohydrates, making grains important for heart health. In addition, most grain products are excellent sources of B vitamins and iron, and whole grain products are good sources of fiber. Choices include:

Breads

bagel	½ small
biscuit†	1 small
bread, sandwich	1 slice
cornbread, 2-inch square†	1
English muffin	½
muffin	1 medium
roll, dinner	1 small
frankfurter	½
hamburger	½
hard	½ medium
tortilla, corn	1 6-inch
pita pocket	1 small

Cereals & Pasta

barley, corn, oats, rice, wheat cereals	
cold	1 ounce or ¾ cup
hot, cooked	½ cup
uncooked	¼ cup
bran cereal	⅓ cup
pasta or noodles, cooked	½ cup
wheat germ	¼ cup
whole grain kernels	
barley, buckwheat groats, bulgur,	

34

grits, hominy, rice, cooked	½ cup
popcorn, air-popped	2 cups

Crackers

arrowroot	3
breadsticks, 5-inches long, ½-inch wide	3
flatbread, thin wafers	4
graham, 2½-inch squares	2
melba toast, rectangular	5
round	6
oyster	20
saltines	6
whole grain, 2 by 3½-inches	3

Baking Ingredients

arrowroot	2 tablespoons
bread crumbs, dry	3 tablespoons
cornmeal	2 tablespoons
cornstarch	2 tablespoons
flour	2 tablespoons
tapioca	2 tablespoons

Vegetables

corn, whole kernel	⅓ cup
on cob	1 small
potato, white, whole	1 small
mashed	½ cup
sweet potato (yam), whole	½ small
mashed	¼ cup

†Omit 1 fat group unit
All values are for products without added salt or fat.

LEGUMES

Legumes are good sources of protein, yet contain virtually no cholesterol or fat. At the same time, they provide an abundance of complex carbohydrates, fiber, vitamins, and minerals. Due to their heart-healthy characteristics, legumes should be liberally included in the diet. Choices include:

Dried beans	½ cup

black
Great Northern
kidney
lima
mung
navy
pinto
white

Dried peas	½ cup

black-eyed
chick (garbanzo)
cow
split

Lentils	½ cup

MEAT AND ALTERNATIVES

Besides providing substantial amounts of protein, this group contributes B vitamins, iron, and phosphorus to your diet. Since most animal products are high in cholesterol and saturated fat, use the purchasing and cooking tips in Chapter IV, along with Appendices A, B, and C, to assist you in making heart-healthy food decisions.

Accordingly, meat and alternatives are classified according to fat content. Choices include:

Very Low-Fat

chicken, without skin	1 ounce
Cornish hen, without skin	1 ounce
cottage cheese, dry	¼ cup
egg whites	2
fish: bluefish, cod, flounder, halibut,	1 ounce
herring, red snapper, sardines,	
smelt, sole, striped bass,	

swordfish, whiting
pheasant, without skin	1 ounce
tuna, packed in water	1 ounce
turkey, without skin	1 ounce
shellfish	
clams, shrimp, oyster	5 small
lobster	1 ounce

Moderately Low-Fat

beef: chipped, flank steak, tenderloin	1 ounce
cheese:	
with less than 5 percent animal fat††	1 ounce
cottage cheese, creamed	¼ cup
mozzarella, part-skim	1 ounce
Parmesan	3 tablespoons
duck, without skin	1 ounce
fish: bass, carp, salmon, trout, whitefish	1 ounce
lamb: leg, rib, roast, shank	1 ounce
pork: leg, shoulder, tenderloin	1 ounce
tofu	3 ounces
tuna, packed in oil	1 ounce
veal: cutlets, leg, loin, rib, shank, shoulder	1 ounce

††To calculate the percentage of fat in one serving (1 ounce or 28 grams), use the information on the product label and divide grams of fat in 1 serving (1 ounce) by 28 grams, then multiply by 100.
For example: 7 grams fat/serving divided by 28 grams = .25
$$.25 \times 100 = 25\% \text{ fat content}$$

MILK PRODUCTS

In addition to legumes and meat and alternatives, milk products are good sources of protein. However, unlike legumes and like meat and alternatives, some milk products are high in saturated fat. For this reason, choose low-fat milk products for heart health.

Most milk products are excellent sources of calcium, a nutrient important for the development and maintenance of strong bones and teeth at *all* ages. Fortified milk is also a good source of vitamins A and D. Choices include:

Very Low-Fat

buttermilk, made from skim milk	1 cup
evaporated low-fat milk, undiluted	½ cup
non-fat dry milk, undiluted	¼ cup
skim milk	1 cup
yogurt, plain (made with non-fat milk)	1 cup

Moderately Low-Fat

buttermilk, made from whole milk	1 cup
low-fat milk, 1%	1 cup
yogurt, plain (made with low-fat milk)	1 cup

NOTE: Buttermilk can be a significant source of sodium. Limit your intake of this if so advised by your doctor or dietitian. Some companies are now producing low-salt buttermilk. Ask your grocery store manager if you cannot find it.

FATS

Since the individual ratio of polyunsaturated, mono-unsaturated, and saturated fats in the diet is crucial to heart health, they are classified as such. Choices include:

Polyunsaturated:

avocado	⅛ small
margarine, tub (made with polyunsaturated oil)	1 teaspoon
oils, vegetable (except coconut, olive, palm, and peanut)	1 teaspoon
olives	5 small
nuts (except Brazil, cashews, macadamia, and pistachio)	5
mayonnaise	2 teaspoons
salad dressings, except those containing cheese	2 teaspoons
seeds: pumpkin, sunflower	1 tablespoon

Monounsaturated:

margarine, liquid or stick (made with polyunsaturated oil)	1 teaspoon
oils: olive, peanut	1 teaspoon

SUGARS

honey	2½ teaspoons
jam	1 tablespoon
jelly	1 tablespoon
maple syrup	1 tablespoon
molasses	1 tablespoon
sugar	1 tablespoon

FREE FOODS

Aromatic bitters
Coffee
Herbs and spices, with no added salt or sodium
Seltzer or mineral water
Tea

COUNTING CALORIES

Not only do different people have different personalities, but they also have different caloric needs. These caloric requirements are based on body size, height, age, sex, and activity level. To determine your personal caloric requirement to achieve or maintain ideal weight, refer to the following guidelines.

1. Calculate your basal caloric requirements (the energy you expend at rest) by multiplying your personal weight goal or your ideal weight (see Table IIIC) by one of the following factors:

Age	Women	Men
under 45	10	11
over 45	9	10

2. Adjust caloric requirements for age by subtracting 10 calories for each year over 25 from your basal energy requirement.
3. Add calories for physical activity by multiplying the figure derived in guideline 2 by one of the following:
   • sedentary (office work) = .3
   • moderately sedentary (occasional participation in an exercise program) = .4
   • moderately active (participation in a regular exercise program) = .5
   • extremely active (Olympic hopeful) = 1

For example, using the formula above and Table IIIC, a woman with the following characteristics—47 years of age, small frame, 5 feet 4 inches tall, and sedentary—would calculate her caloric requirements as indicated below:

1. 140 pounds × 9 calories/pound = 1260 calories
2. 47 years − 25 years = 22 years
   22 years × 10 calories/year = 220 calories
   1260 calories − 220 calories = 1040 calories
3. 1040 calories × .3 = 312 calories
   1040 + 312 = 1352 total calories

As you can see, the less active you are, the fewer calories you can afford to eat without gaining weight.

To help you either achieve or maintain your ideal weight in a heart-healthy manner, we provide suggested diet plans for 1600 and 2000 calories, which are low in fat and high in complex carbohydrates. Both diets use the Heart Smart Plan food groups for guidance in choosing the proper kinds and amounts of foods.

If your calorie requirements are different, follow these easy steps to meet your own needs:

1. Refer to the food group units that correspond to the calorie level closest to your own requirements.
2. Calculate your food group units on a ratio basis.
   For example, a person who requires 1850 calories would follow these steps:

40

a. Refer to the food group units that correspond to 2000 calories.
b. Multiply all food group units by 1850/2000 or 0.9250 (4 fruit group units × 0.9250 = 3¾ fruit group units).
c. It may be impractical to reduce servings by ¼ of a food group unit, so it would be necessary to calculate as instructed, then adjust food group units as practical. For example, for 1850 calories, you may want to keep 4 fruit group units, but will choose to reduce vegetable group units to 4, even though when figured on a ratio basis, you would be allowed 4½ vegetables.

GOVERNING GUIDELINES

In order to increase your chances of success in reducing your risk for developing coronary heart disease, follow these tips:

1. Consult your physician.
2. Monitor your eating and activity behaviors by utilizing the information in Chapter II.
3. Familiarize yourself with foods that contain small or large amounts of cholesterol, fats, and sodium. (See Appendices A, B, and C.)
4. Follow the suggested food group units for a diet of 1600 or 2000 calories, or calculate your own individual energy needs.
5. Study the sample menus that follow to assist you in designing your own diet.

MENU MAGIC

The following menus show how you can use the Heart Smart Plan food groups and diets to plan tasty, satisfying meals for the day. For your convenience, we've given you two weekday menus and one weekend menu, suitable for entertaining. Recipes for the asterisked (*) items are found in Chapter V. Your guests will appreciate your concern for their health, too.

You will see that the total servings of food groups each day do not exactly match the diets for 1600 and 2000 calories provided on the previous page. The menus have been de-

Table IIIC
HEIGHT AND WEIGHT TABLE

Height Feet	Inches	Men Small Frame	Medium Frame	Large Frame	Height Feet	Inches	Women Small Frame	Medium Frame	Large Frame
5	2	128–134	131–141	138–150	4	10	102–111	109–121	118–131
5	3	130–136	133–143	140–153	4	11	103–113	111–123	120–134
5	4	132–138	135–145	142–156	5	0	104–115	113–126	122–137
5	5	134–140	137–148	144–160	5	1	106–118	115–129	125–140
5	6	136–142	139–151	146–164	5	2	108–121	118–132	128–143
5	7	138–145	142–154	149–168	5	3	111–124	121–135	131–147
5	8	140–148	145–157	152–172	5	4	114–127	124–138	134–151
5	9	142–151	148–160	155–176	5	5	117–130	127–141	137–155
5	10	144–154	151–163	158–180	5	6	120–133	130–144	140–159
5	11	146–157	154–166	161–184	5	7	123–136	133–147	143–163
6	0	149–160	157–170	164–188	5	8	126–139	136–150	146–167
6	1	152–164	160–174	168–192	5	9	129–142	139–153	149–170
6	2	155–168	164–178	172–197	5	10	132–145	142–156	152–173
6	3	158–172	167–182	176–202	5	11	135–148	145–159	155–176
6	4	162–176	171–187	181–207	6	0	138–151	148–162	158–179

Weights, at ages 25–59 based on lowest mortality, given in pounds according to frame (in indoor clothing weighing 5 pounds for men and 3 pounds for women; shoes with 1"-heels).

Source: Metropolitan Life Insurance Company, Health and Safety Division, 1983.

signed this way to show you that it is not necessary to follow the plans *exactly*. What is important is that you generally eat as suggested, paying more attention to the types of food you eat and the way the foods are prepared, rather than exact amounts. Of course, this does not mean you should eat more than suggested if you are trying to lose weight, or if you find you are gaining undesired weight. Use your common sense in these matters.

Food Group	1600 calories	2000 calories
Vegetables	4 units	5 units
Fruit	4 units	4 units
Grains	6 units	8 units
Legumes	½ unit	1 unit
Meat and Alternatives*		
Very Low-Fat	–	1 unit
Moderately Low-Fat	3 units	3 units
Milk Products*		
Very Low-Fat	2 units	1 unit
Moderately Low-Fat	–	1 unit
Fats		
Polyunsaturated	4 units	5 units
Monounsaturated	3 units	4 units
Sugars	2 units	2 units

*NOTE: If the higher fat categories are designated, it is acceptable to choose foods from the lower-fat categories. However, it is not appropriate to choose more food group units than suggested from the higher-fat categories, unless that choice is adjusted for by choosing lower-fat categories in other groups. (See example on Sample Menu Day 1, 1600 calories where very low-fat meats are chosen and 1 moderately low-fat milk is chosen.)

THE HEART SMART 1600 CALORIE FOOD PLAN SAMPLE WEEKDAY MENU 1

FOOD GROUPS	BREAKFAST	FOR 2000 CALORIES CHANGE AMOUNTS AS FOLLOWS:
2 Fruit	⅔ cup chilled apple juice mixed with	
Free Food	Sparkling mineral water and served over ice	
2 Grains	1 small toasted sesame-seed bagel spread with	
2 Fats, Polyunsaturated	2 teaspoons tub margarine and	
1 Sugar	1 tablespoon raspberry preserves	
Free Food	Hot coffee or tea	

LUNCH

2 Vegetables	1 serving Pasta and Vegetable Salad*	
1 Grain		
1 Fat, Polyunsaturated		
1 Grain	1 small crusty roll, warmed	2 medium crusty rolls, warmed (Adds 1 Grain)
1 Fruit	1 serving Berry Frost*	
1 Milk Product, Very Low-Fat		
½ Sugar		

DINNER

½ Legumes	1 serving Bean Dip* with	2 servings Bean Dip* (Adds ½ Legume)
1 Vegetable	½ cup fresh carrot sticks	1 cup fresh carrot sticks (Adds 1 Vegetable)
1 Vegetable	1 serving Mexican Baked Fish*	
1 Grain		
3½ Meat and Alternatives, Very Low-Fat		
1 Grain	½ cup fluffy brown rice with	1 cup fluffy brown rice (Adds 1 Grain)
2 Fats, Monounsaturated	onions sauteed in 2 teaspoons olive oil	
½ Sugar	1 serving Mocha Meringues*	

SNACK

1 Fruit	1 chilled fresh pear, sliced and topped with	
1 Milk Product, Moderately Low-Fat	1 cup low-fat plain yogurt sprinkled with	
1 Fat, Polyunsaturated	1 tablespoon sunflower seeds	2 tablespoons sunflower seeds (Adds 1 Fat, Polyunsaturated)

TOTAL SERVINGS OF FOOD GROUPS FOR DAY 1:

1600 Calorie Menu:	2000 Calorie Menu:
4 Vegetables	5 Vegetables
4 Fruits	4 Fruits
6 Grains	8 Grains
½ Legume	1 Legume
3½ Meat and Alternatives, Very Low-Fat	3½ Meat and Alternatives, Very Low-Fat
2 Milk Products, 1 Very Low-Fat 1 Moderately Low-Fat	2 Milk Products, 1 Very Low-Fat 1 Moderately Low-Fat
6 Fats, 4 Polyunsaturated 2 Monounsaturated	7 Fats, 5 Polyunsaturated 2 Monounsaturated
2 Sugars	2 Sugars

FOOD GROUPS	BREAKFAST	FOR 2000 CALORIES CHANGE AMOUNTS AS FOLLOWS:
1 Grain	1 oven-warmed Honey Bran Muffin*	2 Honey Bran Muffins* (Adds 1 Grain, 1 Fat, Polyunsaturated)
2 Fats, Polyunsaturated	spread with 2 teaspoons tub margarine	4 teaspoons tub margarine (Adds 2 Fats, Polyunsaturated)
1 Sugar	1 tablespoon orange marmalade	
1 Milk Product, Very Low-Fat	1 cup ice-cold skim milk	
1 Fruit	½ cup melon in season with lime slice	

LUNCH

2 Vegetables	1 serving Split Pea Soup*	
1 Legume		
1 Fat, Polyunsaturated		
1 Meat and Alternatives, Very Low-Fat	Deviled Chicken in Endive*	
2 Grains	6 low-fat, low-sodium whole-grain crackers	
3 Fruits	1 cup unsweetened pineapple juice	

DINNER

2 Vegetables	1 serving Veal and Peppers*	
3 Meat and Alternatives, Very Low-Fat		
1 Vegetable	1 serving Orzo Salad*	
1 Grain		
2 Fats, Monounsaturated		
1 Grain	1 slice Italian bread	2 slices Italian bread (Adds 1 Grain) 1 teaspoon stick margarine (Adds 1 Fat, Monounsaturated)

SNACK

1 Milk Product, Very Low-Fat	1 cup skim milk flavored with
Free Food	¼ teaspoon vanilla extract and
½ Sugar	1 teaspoon sugar
1 Grain	2 squares graham crackers

TOTAL SERVINGS OF FOOD GROUPS FOR DAY 2:

1600 Calorie Menu:	2000 Calorie Menu:
5 Vegetables	5 Vegetables
4 Fruits	4 Fruits
6 Grains	8 Grains
1 Legume	1 Legume
4 Meat and Alternatives,	4 Meat and Alternatives,
1 Very Low-Fat	1 Very Low-Fat
3 Moderately Low-Fat	3 Moderately Low-Fat
2 Milk Products, Very Low-Fat	2 Milk Products, Very Low-Fat
5 Fats,	9 Fats,
3 Polyunsaturated	6 Polyunsaturated
2 Monounsaturated	3 Monounsaturated
1½ Sugars	1½ Sugars

THE HEART SMART 1600 CALORIE FOOD PLAN SAMPLE WEEKEND MENU

FOOD GROUPS	BRUNCH	FOR 2000 CALORIES CHANGE AMOUNTS AS FOLLOWS
1 Fruit	½ pink grapefruit with mint sprig	
1 Fruit	1 serving Whole Wheat Pancakes with Rosy	2 Servings Whole Wheat
1½ Grains	Applesauce* with	Pancakes with Rosy Applesauce
1 Fat, Polyunsaturated		(Adds 1 Fruit, 1½ Grains, 1 Fat, Polyunsaturated)
1 Sugar	1 tablespoon maple syrup and	2 tablespoons maple syrup (Adds 1 Sugar)
2 Fats, Monounsaturated	2 teaspoons stick margarine	4 teaspoons stick margarine (Adds 2 Fats, Monounsaturated)
1 Milk Product, Very Low-Fat	1 cup ice-cold skim milk	
Free Food	Hot coffee or tea	

MIDAFTERNOON SNACK

½ Vegetable	½ serving Three Bean Casserole*	
¾ Legume		
2 Grains	6 small bread sticks	

DINNER

1 Vegetable	1 serving Egg Drop Soup*	
2 Vegetables	1 serving Beef Chop Suey*	
1½ Grains		
3 Meat and Alternatives, Moderately Low-Fat		
2 Vegetables	1 serving Snow Peas and Water Chestnuts*	
1 Fat, Polyunsaturated		
2 Fruits	1 cup chilled fresh melon in season	
Free Food	Chinese tea	

EVENING SNACK

1 Fruit	1 serving Curried Fruit and Nuts*	
2 Fats, Polyunsaturated		
1 Milk Product, Very Low-Fat	1 serving Irish Coffee Milk Shake*	
1 Sugar		

TOTAL SERVINGS OF FOOD GROUPS FOR WEEKEND:

1600 Calorie Menu:	2000 Calorie Menu:
5½ Vegetables	5½ Vegetables
5 Fruits	5 Fruits
5 Grains	6½ Grains
¾ Legume	1 Legume
3 Meat and Alternatives, Moderately Low-Fat	4 Meat and Alternatives, 1 Very Low-Fat 3 Moderately Low-Fat
2 Milk Products, Very Low-Fat	2 Milk Products, Very Low-Fat
6 Fats, 4 Polyunsaturated 2 Monounsaturated	9 Fats, 5 Polyunsaturated 4 Monounsaturated
2 Sugars	3 Sugars

CHAPTER IV

FROM READING LABELS TO SETTING TABLES

In preceding chapters, you learned how to change your eating and exercise habits to better your heart health. This chapter takes you further with tips on choosing and preparing foods. Specifically, it covers:

- How to modify recipes
- How to prepare heart-healthy foods
- How to shop for food
- How to choose foods in a variety of social situations

MODIFYING RECIPES FOR HEART HEALTH

Try these easy-to-follow techniques and tips for modifying and preparing your own family favorites. By using the suggested substitutions, you can significantly lower the cholesterol, fat and sodium content of standard recipes.

FOR	SUBSTITUTE
• sour cream	• low-fat yogurt
• creamed cottage cheese (4% fat)	• low-fat cottage cheese (1% fat), pot cheese, farmer's cheese

• ricotta cheese	• part-skim ricotta cheese
• heavy cream	• evaporated, skim or low-fat milk
• whole milk	• low-fat milk (1–2% fat), skim milk
• butter	• margarine made with liquid vegetable oil
• oil	• corn or safflower oil
• salad dressings	• yogurt mixed with mustard, lemon, herbs and spices, or oil-free dressings
• luncheon meats	• turkey and chicken breast
• tuna packed in oil	• tuna packed in water
• red meat protein sources	• dried peas and beans (legumes), pasta, grains, cereals
• potato chips, corn chips	• salt-free pretzels, air-popped popcorn
• chocolate candies	• dried fruits, nuts (except Brazil, cashews, macadamia and pistachio), sesame and sun-flower seeds
• ice cream, ice milk	• sherbet
• commercial gravies	• homemade gravies, skimmed of fat
• self-basting turkey	• regular turkey, basted
• prime or choice grades of meat	• good or standard grades of meat
• hard cheeses: cheddar, Swiss, Muenster	• Swiss-Chris, part-skim mozzarella
• chocolate cake	• angel food cake
• pastries	• bran muffins, graham crackers
• 1 cup solid shortening	• ⅔ cup polyunsaturated vegetable oil
• 1 egg	• 2 egg whites
• cooking vegetables in butter	• steam vegetables; flavor with herbs
• biscuits, muffins, croissants	• hard rolls, pita pockets, Italian bread, sandwich bread
• high-fat crackers	• bread sticks, graham crackers, whole grain crackers, melba toast
• sautéing foods in fat	• sauté in non-stick skillet without oil or use skillet sprayed with non-stick cooking spray

• browning meats in fat	• brown in its own fat
• preparing gravies	• chill until fat congeals and lift off fat, or dip paper towel in gravy to absorb fat, or use a gravy skimmer
• cooking poultry	• remove skin, then cook as recipe directs
• cooking meats	• trim all visible fat from meat prior to cooking; cook on a rack to drain fat
• buttering breads, muffins, and vegetables	• dip a pastry brush in sesame oil and lightly paint breads, muffins, and vegetables
• commercial tenderizers	• tenderize with a meat mallet and a homemade marinade
• poaching meat, fish, and poultry in cream sauce	• use vegetable stock or clear broth
• purchasing beef	• choose lean cuts: loin, chuck, ground beef, flank steak
• purchasing pork	• choose lean cuts: pork pieces, arm roast, loin
• purchasing lamb	• choose lean cuts: leg, loin, rib, shoulder
• purchasing veal	• choose lean cuts: cutlets, sirloin roast, veal breast

SUPERMARKET SURVIVAL

It's often said that healthful eating takes too much time in planning and shopping and costs too much for the average budget. But don't believe it. Healthful eating can be accomplished easily and within a budget by following many of the guidelines below.

- Plan menus; then make a list to enable you to recall all necessary heart-healthy grocery items. Recipe preparation goes much faster when you have all necessary ingredients on hand.
- Take an inventory to avoid buying foods in duplicate and thereby spending more than needed.
- Eat before you shop to avoid impulse buying of non-heart healthy foods.

- Use coupons and comparison shop to save money.
- Buy store brands or no frills to economize on heart-healthy foods.
- Choose larger quantity sizes, if your food storage space allows.
- Read labels to become familiar with the products you buy and eat. The information on labels can help you take advantage of specials by telling you whether the food will fit into your diet.

In reading the ingredient list on food labels, you may come across a number of words that are unfamiliar. Some of these "foreign" words should become familiar to you. For example, although a number of ingredients do not contain the word "fat" in their names, they are in fact high in fat content, particularly saturated fat. Such ingredient names include:

- glycerol
- hydrogenated shortening
- lard
- coconut and coconut oil
- palm oil

Any ingredients which contain the word "sodium" should also be noted. The more mention there is of sodium or undesirable fats, the more likely the food should be avoided. Ask your doctor or dietitian for advice about a particular food if you are not certain. The order in which ingredients appear is also important. Listed by weight, an ingredient that appears at the beginning of the list is the ingredient in greatest quantity.

SOCIAL SITUATION SAVVY

Do you feel your busy schedule doesn't allow you to follow heart-healthy guidelines? Do you seem to have less control over your food choices at social occasions? Help is on the way. It *is* possible to diet in all social situations. But remember, no one can do it for you; you must do it for yourself. Make these promises to yourself to optimize your social situation savvy:

- Be aggressive. Do not allow people to talk you into eating foods you know you shouldn't have.

- Eat a light meal or snack before attending a special function where food is plentiful. By fasting before such a gathering, you tend to eat too much.
- Do not feel obligated to join the "clean plate club." Rid yourself of food guilt; you will be doing yourself a favor by helping to make your heart healthy.
- In restaurants, follow the same guidelines for choosing foods as you would in your own home. When ordering any foods, always request dressings, gravies, and other condiments on the side to enable you to control portion sizes. Be aggressive, and be honest with yourself.
- If you cannot possibly turn down a favorite dessert, eat only half.
- Keep talking. The more your mouth is involved in conversation, the less it is involved in eating.
- Choose raw or steamed vegetables to increase your fiber and complex carbohydrate intake. Balance, variety, and moderation are the basic keys to healthier living. Do it today for yourself, and you will be helping to make your heart healthier for today and tomorrow.

In an ideal world, television commercials would urge Americans to eat not junk diets, but nutritious diets. Vending machines would contain fruit juices and nutritious snacks, rather than sugary soft drinks and fatty candy bars. Labels on all processed foods would boldly state fat, sugar, and salt content. Restaurants specializing in low-cholesterol cuisine would become fashionable all over the country.

As you know, it's a far from perfect world. But you're learning to reevaluate your part of it to suit yourself and the needs of your increasingly healthy body.

CHAPTER V

RECIPES FOR A MORE HEALTHY HEART

The Heart Smart recipes do more than show you how to put the plan into action. They're tasty and sure to satisfy the whole family. With them, it is easy to plan a diet, not only for the person in your household who has been diagnosed as needing cholesterol reduction, but also for the rest of the family. Try them and enjoy good eating for your heart's health!

Appetizers

Deviled Chicken in Endive

¾ cup chopped, cooked
  chicken (6 ounces raw or 5
  ounces cooked)
2 tablespoons plain low-fat
  yogurt

1 tablespoon finely chopped
   green onion
1 teaspoon mayonnaise
1 teaspoon dry mustard
⅛ teaspoon salt
⅛ teaspoon pepper
8 Belgian endive leaves

In small bowl, combine chicken, yogurt, green onion, mayonnaise, mustard, salt, and pepper. Cover and refrigerate about 1 hour. Before serving, spoon an equal amount of mixture on wide end of endive leaf. Sprinkle with chopped parsley, if desired. Makes 8 servings.

Approximate Nutrient Analysis Per Serving:
Calories: 40
Protein: 5 grams
Fat: 2 grams
Carbohydrate: 0
Cholesterol: 16 milligrams
Sodium: 55 milligrams
Potassium: 60 milligrams

Food Group Units:
Meat and Alternatives:
      Very Low-Fat: 1

Curried Fruit and Nuts

40 whole blanched almonds
   (⅓ cup)
24 walnut halves (½ cup)
¾ cup raisins, plumped in
   water
2 tablespoons margarine
1 teaspoon curry powder
⅛ teaspoon ground red
   pepper

Preheat oven to 325°F.
In medium bowl, combine almonds, walnuts, and drained raisins.

In small saucepan over low heat, melt margarine. Add curry and red pepper; cook about 1 minute, stirring frequently. Pour over nut mixture; toss well.

On baking pan sprayed with non-stick cooking spray, spread mixture. Bake about 15–20 minutes, or until nuts are lightly browned, stirring occasionally. Spread on wax paper to cool. May be served warm or at room temperature. Makes 8 servings, about ¼ cup each.

Approximate Nutrient Analysis Per Serving:
Calories: 150
Protein: 3 grams
Fat: 11 grams
Carbohydrate: 13 grams
Cholesterol: 0
Sodium: 35 milligrams
Potassium: 180 milligrams

Food Group Units:
Fruit: 1
Fat:
    Polyunsaturated: 2

Eggplant Caviar

2 tablespoons vegetable oil
2 cups finely chopped
   eggplant (¾–1 pound,
   untrimmed)
¼ cup finely chopped onion
2 garlic cloves, minced
2 medium tomatoes, peeled
   and chopped (1 cup)
1½ tablespoons fresh lemon
   juice
½ teaspoon oregano, crushed
½ teaspoon ground cumin
¼ teaspoon salt
⅛ teaspoon pepper
unsalted whole grain crackers

54

In large non-stick skillet over high heat in hot vegetable oil, cook eggplant, onion, and garlic about 5 minutes or until soft, stirring occasionally. Add remaining ingredients, except crackers; cover. Cook about 20–25 minutes, stirring occasionally. Transfer to small bowl; cover. Refrigerate about 1 hour. Serve with crackers. Makes 8 servings, about ¼ cup each.

Approximate Nutrient Analysis Per Serving:
Calories: 50
Protein: 1 gram
Fat: 4 grams
Carbohydrate: 4 grams
Cholesterol: 70 milligrams
Sodium: 0
Potassium: 130 milligrams

Food Group Units:
Vegetables: 1
Fat:
   Polyunsaturated: ½

Stuffed Cherry Tomatoes

16 cherry tomatoes (½ pint
   container)
1 3¼-ounce can tuna in water,
   drained and flaked (¾ cup)
2 tablespoons plain low-fat
   yogurt
2 teaspoons finely chopped
   green onion
2 teaspoons chili sauce
¼ teaspoon prepared
   horseradish
⅛ teaspoon pepper

With a sharp knife, slice tops of tomatoes. With a grape-fruit spoon, remove pulp; drain upside down on paper towels.

In small bowl, combine remaining ingredients. Spoon an equal amount into tomatoes. Refrigerate about 1 hour. Makes 4 servings.

Approximate Nutrient Analysis Per Serving:
Calories: 35
Protein: 6 grams
Fat: 0
Carbohydrate: 3 grams
Cholesterol: 12 milligrams
Sodium: 125 milligrams
Potassium: 160 milligrams

Food Group Units:
Vegetables: ½
Meat and Alternatives:
    Very Low-Fat: ½

Mexican Cheese Dip

1 cup plain low-fat yogurt
½ cup low-fat cottage cheese
2 tablespoons margarine
1 garlic clove, minced
2 tablespoons chopped green
  chilies
1 teaspoon chili powder
⅛ teaspoon pepper

In small bowl, combine all ingredients. Cover and refrigerate about 1 hour. Stir well before serving. Serve with assorted fresh vegetables. Makes 6 servings, about ½ cup each.

Approximate Nutrient Analysis Per Serving:
Calories: 75
Protein: 4
Fat: 1.5
Carbohydrate: 6
Cholesterol: 3 milligrams
Sodium: 150 milligrams
Potassium: 115 milligrams

Food Group Units:
Meat and Alternatives:

Moderately Low-Fat: ½
Fat:
Polyunsaturated: ½

Mushroom Pâté

2 tablespoons margarine
¼ cup finely chopped onion
  (½ small)
¼ cup finely chopped green
  pepper
1 garlic clove, minced
½ cup low-fat cottage cheese
2 eggs
1 pound mushrooms, finely
  chopped
¾ cup plain dry bread crumbs
½ teaspoon salt
½ teaspoon basil, crushed
½ teaspoon oregano, crushed
¼ teaspoon thyme, crushed
⅛ teaspoon pepper

Preheat oven to 325°F.
In small skillet over medium-high heat, melt margarine.
Add onion, green pepper, and garlic; cook, about 4 minutes
or until soft, stirring frequently; set aside.
In large bowl with mixer at medium speed, beat cottage
cheese and eggs until smooth. Stir in remaining ingredients
and onion mixture until well combined. Spoon into pan
sprayed with non-stick cooking spray. Bake 1½–2 hours or
until firm to touch. Cool on wire rack 30 minutes. Remove
from pan. Cover and refrigerate overnight. Makes 10 servings.

Approximate Nutrient Analysis Per Serving:
Calories: 90
Protein: 5 grams
Fat: 4 grams
Carbohydrate: 9 grams
Cholesterol: 55 milligrams

Sodium: 260 milligrams
Potassium: 245 milligrams

Food Group Units:
Vegetables: 1
Grains: ½
Fat:
    Polyunsaturated: 1

Pita Crisps

2 small whole wheat pita
  pocket breads
4 teaspoons margarine,
  melted
½ teaspoon oregano, crushed
⅛ teaspoon thyme, crushed
⅛ teaspoon garlic powder
1 teaspoon poppy seeds

Preheat oven to 400°F.
Split each pita bread in half. Cut each half into 8 triangles.
In small bowl, combine margarine, oregano, thyme, and garlic powder; brush evenly over each pita triangle; place on baking sheet. Sprinkle with poppy seeds. Bake about 10–15 minutes or until crisp. Makes 4 servings.

Approximate Nutrient Analysis Per Serving:
Calories: 115
Protein: 3 grams
Fat: 5 grams
Carbohydrate: 15 grams
Cholesterol: 0
Sodium: 45 milligrams
Potassium: 12 milligrams

Food Group Units:
Grains: 1
Fat:
    Polyunsaturated: 1

Bean Dip

1 8¾-ounce can kidney beans,
   drained and rinsed
2 tablespoons minced onion
1 clove garlic, minced
1 tablespoon yogurt
1 teaspoon mayonnaise
2 tablespoons chopped green
   pepper
⅛ teaspoon dry mustard
1 teaspoon sugar
2 teaspoons tomato paste
⅛ teaspoon salt

In blender or food processor at medium speed, purée all ingredients until smooth; place in small bowl. Cover and refrigerate about 2 hours. Let stand at room temperature about 20 minutes before serving. Makes 8 servings, about 2 tablespoons each.

Approximate Nutrient Analysis Per Serving:
Calories: 40
Protein: 2 grams
Fat: 1 gram
Carbohydrate: 7 grams
Cholesterol: 45 milligrams
Sodium: 50 milligrams
Potassium: 110 milligrams

Food Group Units:
Legumes: ½

Pizza Potato Skins

4 small baking potatoes,
   washed (1¾ lbs.)
½ cup spaghetti sauce
½ cup shredded part-skim
   mozzarella cheese
   (2 ounces)
½ teaspoon oregano

Preheat oven to 450°F.

With fork, pierce potatoes; place on oven rack. Bake 40–45 minutes or until fork-tender; set aside to cool.

Cut each potato lengthwise into quarters. Remove potato pulp to form small shell, leaving about ¼ inch (reserving pulp for mashing). On baking pan sprayed with non-stick cooking spray, place shells. Spread 1½ teaspoons spaghetti sauce over each potato shell. Sprinkle each with 1½ teaspoons cheese. Sprinkle with oregano. Bake about 15 minutes or until skins are crisp and cheese is lightly browned. Makes 4 servings.

Approximate Nutrient Analysis Per Serving:
Calories: 105
Protein: 6 grams
Fat: 4 grams
Carbohydrate: 14 grams
Cholesterol: 15 milligrams
Sodium: 195 milligrams
Potassium: 15 milligrams

Food Group Units:
Grains: 1
Meat and Alternatives:
    Moderately Low-Fat: ½

Onion Cheese Pie

1 tablespoon margarine
1½ cups thinly sliced onion
    (1 large)
1 garlic clove, minced
1 tablespoon all-purpose flour
4 ounces shredded part-skim
    mozzarella cheese (1 cup)
4 eggs, slightly beaten
1½ cups skim milk
3 tablespoons grated
    Parmesan cheese
⅛ teaspoon salt
⅛ teaspoon pepper
⅛ teaspoon nutmeg

Preheat oven to 375°F.

In large non-stick skillet over medium-high heat in hot margarine, cook onion and garlic about 5–7 minutes or until soft, stirring occasionally. Remove from heat; cool about 15 minutes. Stir in flour. Into 9-inch pie plate or quiche pan sprayed with non-stick cooking spray, spoon onion mixture. Sprinkle mozzarella cheese over onions.

In small bowl, combine remaining ingredients; pour over onions and cheese. Bake about 30 minutes or until knife inserted in center comes out clean. Makes 8 servings.

Approximate Nutrient Analysis Per Serving:
Calories: 130
Protein: 9 grams
Fat: 7 grams
Carbohydrate: 7 grams
Cholesterol: 150 milligrams
Sodium: 215 milligrams
Potassium: 175 milligrams

Food Group Units:
Meat and Alternatives:
    Moderately Low-Fat: 1
Milk Products:
    Moderately Low-Fat: ½

Beverages

Tomato Sizzler

½ cup low-sodium vegetable
    juice cocktail
½ cup crushed ice
½ teaspoon prepared
    horseradish
⅛ teaspoon hot pepper sauce

⅛ teaspoon celery seed
1 celery rib

In blender at low speed, blend all ingredients about 30 seconds. Pour into glass. Garnish with celery rib. Makes 1 serving.

Approximate Nutrient Analysis Per Serving:
Calories: 35
Protein: 2 grams
Fat: 0
Carbohydrate: 7 grams
Cholesterol: 0
Sodium: 80 milligrams
Potassium: 380 milligrams

Food Group Units:
Vegetables: 1

Carrot Pineapple Juice

¾ cup shredded carrots
   (1 large)
½ cup water
1 8-ounce can crushed
   pineapple, packed in
   juice
½ cup crushed ice

In blender at medium speed, blend carrots and water about 1 minute. Strain; return liquid to blender. Add remaining ingredients; blend at low speed until smooth. Pour into two glasses. Makes 2 servings.

Approximate Nutrient Analysis Per Serving:
Calories: 85
Protein: 1 gram
Fat: 0
Carbohydrate: 22 grams
Cholesterol: 0
Sodium: 20 milligrams
Potassium: 280 milligrams

Food Group Units:
Fruit: 2

Berry Frost

¾ cup frozen unsweetened
   strawberries, slightly
   thawed
½ cup plain low-fat yogurt
¼ cup skim milk
1 teaspoon sugar
1 teaspoon vanilla extract
1 ice cube

In covered blender at low speed, blend all ingredients until smooth and frothy; pour into glass. Makes 1 serving.

Approximate Nutrient Analysis Per Serving:
Calories: 160
Protein: 9 grams
Fat: 2 grams
Carbohydrate: 23 grams
Cholesterol: 8 milligrams
Sodium: 110 milligrams
Potassium: 555 milligrams

Food Group Units:
Fruit: 1
Sugars: ½

Coco Banana Shake

½ cup skim milk
½ cup plain low-fat yogurt
½ small ripe banana, mashed
1 teaspoon sugar
½ teaspoon vanilla extract
¼ teaspoon coconut extract
1 ice cube

In covered blender at low speed, blend all ingredients about 30 seconds; pour into glass. Makes 1 serving.

Approximate Nutrient Analysis Per Serving:
Calories: 180
Protein: 11 grams
Fat: 2 grams
Carbohydrate: 29 grams
Cholesterol: 9 milligrams
Sodium: 145 milligrams
Potassium: 650 milligrams

Food Group Units:
Fruit: 1
Milk Products:
    Moderately Low-Fat: 1

Rich Mocha Cocoa

1 cup skim milk
1 cinnamon stick
2 teaspoons unsweetened
  cocoa
2 teaspoons sugar
1 teaspoon instant coffee
  powder
¼ teaspoon vanilla extract

In small saucepan over low heat, cook milk and cinnamon stick about 5 minutes. In small bowl, combine cocoa, sugar, and coffee powder. With a whisk, blend mixture into milk; add vanilla. Cook about 2 minutes, stirring frequently. Remove and discard cinnamon stick; pour into mug. Makes 1 serving.

Approximate Nutrient Analysis Per Serving:
Calories: 135
Protein: 9 grams
Fat: 1 gram
Carbohydrate: 24 grams
Cholesterol: 5 milligrams

Sodium: 130 milligrams
Potassium: 510 milligrams

Food Group Units:
Grains: ½
Milk Products:
    Very Low-Fat: 1

Raspberry Frappe

1½ cups orange juice
½ cup fresh raspberries
1 teaspoon sugar
1 egg white
1 cup crushed ice

In covered blender on high speed, blend orange juice, raspberries, sugar, and egg white about 30 seconds. Gradually add ice, blend until thick and frothy; pour into glasses. Makes 4 servings.

Approximate Nutrient Analysis Per Serving:
Calories: 55
Protein: 2 grams
Fat: 0
Carbohydrate: 13 grams
Cholesterol: 0
Sodium: 15 milligrams
Potassium: 210 milligrams

Food Group Units:
Fruit: 1

Irish Coffee Milkshake

½ cup skim milk
½ cup plain low-fat yogurt
2 teaspoons sugar

1 teaspoon instant coffee
   powder
1 teaspoon Irish whiskey

In blender on low speed, blend all ingredients about 30 seconds. Pour into glass. Makes 1 serving.

Approximate Nutrient Analysis Per Serving:
Calories: 160
Protein: 10 grams
Fat: 2 grams
Carbohydrate: 23 grams
Cholesterol: 10 milligrams
Sodium: 145 milligrams
Potassium: 505 milligrams

Food Group Units:
Fat:
Sugar: 1

Spiced Iced Tea

3 cups cold water
4 tea bags
1½ tablespoons sugar
1 cinnamon stick, broken into
   pieces
2 whole cloves
1 orange slice
ice cubes

In medium saucepan, heat water to boiling. Remove from heat; add remaining ingredients. Cover and let steep about 5–7 minutes. Strain and pour tea into tall glasses filled with ice cubes. Makes 4 servings, about ⅔ cup each.

Approximate Nutrient Analysis Per Serving:
Calories: 25
Protein: 2 grams
Fat: 0
Carbohydrate: 6 grams
Cholesterol: 0

Sodium: 0
Potassium: 10 milligrams

Food Group Units:
Sugar: ½

Soups

Cream of Potato Soup

2 tablespoons margarine
½ cup chopped onion
¼ cup chopped celery
1½ cups diced, peeled
  potatoes (1 large)
1 cup low-sodium chicken
  broth
¼ cup chopped fresh parsley
¼ teaspoon thyme, crushed
¼ teaspoon celery seed
¼ teaspoon salt
⅛ teaspoon pepper
1½ cups skim milk

In medium saucepan over medium-high heat, melt margarine. Add onion and celery; cook about 4 minutes or until soft, stirring frequently. Add potatoes, chicken broth, parsley, thyme, celery seed, salt, and pepper; bring to a boil. Reduce heat; cover. Simmer about 15 minutes or until potatoes are almost tender. Add milk; simmer uncovered about 5 minutes, stirring occasionally.

In blender at medium speed, blend about ¼ of the mixture at a time until smooth. Return to saucepan; heat about 1 minute. Makes 4 servings, about 1 cup each.

Approximate Nutrient Analysis Per Serving:
Calories: 150

Protein: 5 grams
Fat: 6 grams
Carbohydrate: 19 grams
Cholesterol: 2 milligrams
Sodium: 265 milligrams
Potassium: 520 milligrams

Food Group Units:
Grains: 15
Milk Products:
    Very Low-Fat: ½
Fat:
    Polyunsaturated: 1

Corn Chowder

2 tablespoons margarine
¼ cup chopped onion
¼ cup chopped red pepper
1 tablespoon all-purpose flour
2 cups skim milk
1⅓ cup frozen whole kernel
    corn
½ teaspoon salt
¼ teaspoon thyme, crushed
⅛ teaspoon pepper

In medium saucepan over medium-high heat, melt margarine. Add onion and red pepper; cook about 4 minutes or until soft, stirring frequently. Add flour; cook about 1 minute, stirring constantly. Gradually add milk, corn, salt, thyme, and pepper. Reduce heat to low; cook about 5–7 minutes or until slightly thickened and corn is tender. Makes 4 servings, about ⅔ cup each.

Approximate Nutrient Analysis Per Serving:
Calories: 155
Protein: 7 grams
Fat: 6 grams
Carbohydrate: 20 grams
Cholesterol: 2 milligrams

Sodium: 400 milligrams
Potassium: 360 milligrams

Food Group Units:
Vegetables: 1
Grains: ½
Milk Products:
   Very Low-Fat: ½
Fat: —
   Polyunsaturated: 1

Vegetable Soup

1 tablespoon vegetable oil
½ cup chopped onion
2 garlic cloves, minced
1 16-ounce can tomatoes in
   juice, chopped
1 cup low-sodium chicken
   broth
1 cup sliced carrots (about 2
   medium)
1 cup sliced celery
¼ cup chopped fresh parsley
1 teaspoon basil, crushed
¼ teaspoon salt
⅛ teaspoon pepper
1 cup frozen lima beans
½ cup water

In medium saucepan over medium-high heat in hot oil, cook onion and garlic about 3 minutes or until soft, stirring frequently. Add tomatoes in juice, chicken broth, carrots, celery, parsley, basil, salt, and pepper; bring to a boil. Reduce heat; cover. Simmer about 20 minutes. Add lima beans and water; bring to a boil. Reduce heat; simmer about 20 minutes or until beans are tender. Makes 6 servings; about ¾ cup each.

Approximate Nutrient Analysis Per Serving:
Calories: 95

Protein: 4 grams
Fat: 3 grams
Carbohydrate: 15 grams
Cholesterol: 0
Sodium: 265 milligrams
Potassium: 525 milligrams

Food Group Units:
Vegetables: 2
Legumes: ¼
Fat:
    Polyunsaturated: ½

Onion Soup

2 tablespoons margarine
2 cups thinly sliced onions
   (2 medium)
1 tablespoon all-purpose flour
4 cups low-sodium beef broth
¼ teaspoon salt
⅛ teaspoon pepper
4 tablespoons grated
   Parmesan cheese

In large saucepan over low heat, melt margarine. Add onion; cook about 15 minutes, stirring frequently. Add flour; cook about 1 minute, stirring constantly. Add beef broth, salt, and pepper; bring to a boil.

Reduce heat; cover. Simmer about 25 minutes or until onions are very soft, stirring occasionally. Sprinkle with Parmesan cheese. Makes 4 servings, about 1 cup each.

Approximate Nutrient Analysis Per Serving:
Calories: 130
Protein: 4 grams
Fat: 8 grams
Carbohydrate: 12 grams
Cholesterol: 4 milligrams
Sodium: 310 milligrams
Potassium: 220 milligrams

Food Group Units:
Vegetables: 2
Fat:
   Polyunsaturated: 1½

Gazpacho

1 cup fresh whole wheat
   bread crumbs (2 slices)
2 tablespoons red wine
   vinegar
2 tablespoons vegetable oil
2 garlic cloves, minced
1 cup seeded, diced
   cucumber
½ cup diced green pepper
2 tablespoons finely chopped
   green onion
3 cups peeled, seeded,
   chopped tomatoes (5–6)
1 cup tomato juice
⅛ teaspoon pepper

In small bowl, combine bread crumbs, vinegar, oil, and garlic; mix to a smooth paste.

In large bowl, combine remaining ingredients; stir in bread paste until well blended. Cover and refrigerate about 4 hours. Makes 6 servings, about ⅔ cup each.

Approximate Nutrient Analysis Per Serving:
Calories: 100
Protein: 3 grams
Fat: 5 grams
Carbohydrate: 12 grams
Cholesterol: 0
Sodium: 125 milligrams
Potassium: 425 milligrams

Food Group Units:
Vegetables: 1
Grains: ½

Fat:
    Polyunsaturated: 1

Dilled Carrot Bisque

2 cups low-sodium chicken
    broth
2 cups sliced carrots
    (3 medium carrots)
¼ cup chopped fresh parsley
2 tablespoons chopped
    shallots
1 garlic clove, minced
½ teaspoon dill weed
¼ teaspoon salt
⅛ teaspoon pepper
½ cup skim milk

In medium saucepan over medium-high heat, add chicken broth, carrots, parsley, shallots, garlic, dill weed, salt, and pepper; bring to a boil. Reduce heat; cover. Simmer about 30 minutes or until carrots are tender.

In covered blender or food processor at medium speed, blend about ¼ of the mixture at a time until smooth. Return to saucepan; stir in milk and heat about 1 minute. Do not boil. Makes 3 servings, about ¾ cup each.

Approximate Nutrient Analysis Per Serving:
Calories: 60
Protein: 2 grams
Fat: 1 gram
Carbohydrate: 11 grams
Cholesterol: 1 milligram
Sodium: 180 milligrams
Potassium: 355 milligrams

Food Group Units:
Vegetables: 2

Split Pea Soup

2 tablespoons margarine
1 cup chopped carrot
½ cup chopped onion
2 garlic cloves, minced
4½ cups water
1½ cups dry split peas
1 bay leaf
1 tablespoon dry white wine
1 teaspoon white vinegar
½ teaspoon salt
½ teaspoon thyme, crushed
⅛ teaspoon pepper

In large saucepan over medium-high heat, melt margarine. Add carrot, onion, and garlic; cook about 4 minutes or until soft, stirring frequently. Add remaining ingredients; bring to a boil. Reduce heat, cover. Simmer about 1–1¼ hours, stirring occasionally. If soup becomes too thick, add additional water. Remove and discard bay leaf. Makes 6 servings, about ¾ cup each.

Approximate Nutrient Analysis Per Serving:
Calories: 225
Protein: 13 grams
Fat: 4 grams
Carbohydrate: 35 grams
Cholesterol: 0
Sodium: 255 milligrams
Potassium: 545 milligrams

Food Group Units:
Vegetables: 2
Legumes: 1
Fat:
    Polyunsaturated: 1

Chicken and Escarole Soup

½ pound escarole, washed
  (4 cups, packed)

2 teaspoons vegetable oil
⅓ cup chopped onion
2 garlic cloves, minced
4 cups low-sodium chicken
  broth
1½ cups shredded, cooked
  chicken (12 ounces raw or 9
  ounces cooked)
¼ teaspoon salt
¼ teaspoon basil, crushed
⅛ teaspoon pepper
4 tablespoons grated
  Parmesan cheese

Trim escarole and tear into bite-size pieces; set aside.

In medium saucepan over medium-high heat in hot oil, cook onion and garlic about 3 minutes or until soft, stirring frequently. Add chicken broth, chicken, escarole, basil, salt, and pepper; bring to a boil. Reduce heat; cover. Simmer about 5 minutes, stirring occasionally. Sprinkle with Parmesan cheese. Makes 4 servings.

Approximate Nutrient Analysis Per Serving:
Calories: 220
Protein: 22 grams
Fat: 10 grams
Carbohydrate: 9 grams
Cholesterol: 60 milligrams
Sodium: 295 milligrams
Potassium: 470 milligrams

Food Group Units:
Vegetables: 1
Meat and Alternatives:
    Very Low-Fat: 2½
    Moderately Low-Fat: ½
Fat:
    Polyunsaturated: 1

Cream of Artichoke Soup

2 tablespoons margarine

½ cup chopped onion
1 tablespoon all-purpose flour
1½ cups low-sodium chicken
   broth
1 9-ounce package frozen
   artichoke hearts
2 tablespoons sherry
¼ teaspoon thyme, crushed
¼ teaspoon salt
⅛ teaspoon pepper
Dash ground nutmeg
1½ cups skim milk

In medium saucepan over medium-high heat, melt margarine. Add onion; cook about 3 minutes or until soft, stirring
frequently. Add flour; cook about 1 minute, stirring constantly. Gradually add chicken broth, artichokes, sherry, thyme,
salt, pepper, and nutmeg, separating artichokes with fork;
bring to a boil. Reduce heat; cover. Simmer about 15 minutes
or until artichokes are tender. Add milk; simmer uncovered
about 5 minutes.

In covered blender at medium speed, blend about ¼
of the mixture at a time until smooth. Return to saucepan; heat about 1 minute. Makes 4 servings, about 1 cup
each.

Approximate Nutrient Analysis Per Serving:
Calories: 135
Protein: 5 grams
Fat: 7 grams
Carbohydrate: 14 grams
Cholesterol: 2 milligrams
Sodium: 330 milligrams
Potassium: 400 milligrams

Food Group Units:
Vegetables: 1½
Milk Products:
     Very Low-Fat: ½
Fat:
     Polyunsaturated: 1

4 cups low-sodium chicken
  broth, divided
1 cup shredded Chinese
  cabbage
2 tablespoons chopped green
  onion
¼ teaspoon ground ginger
¼ teaspoon salt
Dash pepper
1 tablespoon cornstarch
1 egg white
1 tablespoon water

In medium saucepan, combine 3¾ cups chicken broth, cabbage, green onion, ginger, salt, and pepper; bring to a boil.

In small bowl, combine remaining chicken broth and cornstarch until well blended. Add to saucepan; cook about 5 minutes, stirring occasionally. Beat egg white and water. Pour egg into saucepan slowly, stirring slightly with a fork to form threads. Cook about 1 minute. Makes 4 servings, about 1 cup each.

Approximate Nutrient Analysis Per Serving:
Calories: 55
Protein: 2 grams
Fat: 2 grams
Carbohydrate: 8 grams
Cholesterol: 0
Sodium: 150 milligrams
Potassium: 180 milligrams

Food Group Units:
Vegetables: 1

Main Dishes

Vegetable Pizza

1½ cups whole wheat flour
1 teaspoon active dry yeast
1 teaspoon sugar
⅛ teaspoon salt
½ cup warm water (120–130°F)
1 tablespoon vegetable oil,
  divided
½ pound mushrooms, sliced
  (about 2¾ cups)
⅓ cup chopped onions
1 8-ounce can tomato sauce
1 small green pepper, cut into
  rings
4 ounces shredded part-skim
  mozzarella cheese
1 tablespoon grated Parmesan
  cheese

In medium bowl, combine ¾ cup flour, yeast, sugar, and salt; add water and 2 teaspoons oil. With mixer at low speed, beat until flour is just moistened. Gradually stir in remaining flour to make a soft dough.

Onto lightly floured surface, turn dough; knead about 5 minutes or until smooth and elastic. In greased bowl, place dough, turning over to expose greased portion. Cover with towel; set aside in warm place to rise about 45 minutes or until doubled.

Meanwhile, in large non-stick skillet over medium-high heat in remaining hot oil, cook mushrooms and onion about 5 minutes or until tender, stirring occasionally.

Punch down dough. Form dough to fit 12-inch round pizza

pan sprayed with non-stick cooking spray. Spread tomato sauce over dough. Sprinkle with mushroom-onion mixture. Sprinkle with mozzarella and Parmesan cheeses. Bake about 15–20 minutes or until crust is browned. Makes 8 servings.

Approximate Nutrient Analysis Per Serving:
Calories: 155
Protein: 8 grams
Fat: 5 grams
Carbohydrate: 21 grams
Cholesterol: 9 milligrams
Sodium: 265 milligrams
Potassium: 360 milligrams

Food Group Units:
Vegetables: 1
Grains: 1
Meat and Alternatives:
    Moderately Low-Fat: ½
Fat:
    Polyunsaturated: 1

Pasta and Bean Stew

2 teaspoons vegetable oil
½ cup chopped onion
½ cup chopped green pepper
2 garlic cloves, minced
1 16-ounce can tomatoes in
    juice, chopped
1 cup small pasta shells
    (4 ounces dry)
1 cup water
½ teaspoon oregano, crushed
¼ teaspoon basil, crushed
⅛ teaspoon pepper
1 16-ounce can chick peas
    (garbanzo beans), drained
    and rinsed
1 8¾-ounce can kidney beans,
    undrained

1 tablespoon grated Parmesan
  cheese

In medium saucepan over medium-high heat in hot oil,
cook onion, green pepper, and garlic about 3 minutes or until
soft. Add tomatoes in juice; bring to a boil. Add pasta, water,
oregano, basil, and pepper; reduce heat. Cover; simmer
about 10 minutes or until pasta is tender, stirring occasionally. Rinse kidney beans, reserving liquid. Add chick peas,
kidney beans with liquid, and cheese; cook about 5 minutes
or until heated through, stirring frequently. Makes 6 servings,
about ¾ cup each.

Approximate Nutrient Analysis Per Serving:
Calories: 215
Protein: 10 grams
Fat: 3 grams
Carbohydrate: 37 grams
Cholesterol: 0
Sodium: 260 milligrams
Potassium: 510 milligrams

Food Group Units:
Vegetables: 1
Grains: 1
Legumes: 1

Rice and Pasta Medley

1 tablespoon margarine
½ cup chopped onion
½ cup chopped celery
½ cup brown rice
2 ounces vermicelli, broken
  up (¾ cup)
1¼ cups low-sodium chicken
  broth
½ cup water
¼ cup dry white wine
¼ teaspoon salt
½ teaspoon thyme, crushed

⅛ teaspoon pepper
¼ cup chopped fresh parsley

In large non-stick skillet over medium-high heat in hot margarine, cook onion and celery about 3 minutes or until soft, stirring occasionally. Add rice and vermicelli; cook until lightly browned, stirring occasionally. Add remaining ingredients, except parsley; bring to a boil. Reduce heat; cover. Simmer about 30–40 minutes or until rice is tender, stirring occasionally. Stir in parsley. Makes 6 servings, about ½ cup each.

Approximate Nutrient Analysis Per Serving:
Calories: 125
Protein: 3 grams
Fat: 3 grams
Carbohydrate: 2 grams
Cholesterol: 0
Sodium: 105 milligrams
Potassium: 320 milligrams

Food Group Units:
Vegetables: 1
Grains: 1
Fat:
    Polyunsaturated: ½

Spinach Stuffed Shells

1 10-ounce package frozen
   chopped spinach, thawed
   and well drained
4 ounces part-skim ricotta
   cheese (½ cup)
2 ounces shredded part-skim
   mozzarella cheese (½ cup)
1 egg, lightly beaten
1 tablespoon grated Parmesan
   cheese
⅛ teaspoon ground nutmeg
⅛ teaspoon pepper
4 ounces jumbo shells (16)

80

1 15½-ounce jar spaghetti
   sauce

In medium bowl, mix spinach, ricotta and mozzarella cheese, egg, Parmesan cheese, nutmeg, and pepper; set aside.

Cook shells as label directs, omitting salt.

Preheat oven to 350°F.

Fill each shell with about 1 tablespoon of spinach mixture. Into bottom of a 9-inch square baking dish, spoon ½ cup of the spaghetti sauce. Place shells in single layer over sauce. Pour remaining sauce over shells. Bake about 20–30 minutes until heated through and bubbly. Makes 4 servings.

Approximate Nutrient Analysis Per Serving:
Calories: 305
Protein: 16 grams
Fat: 12 grams
Carbohydrate: 37 grams
Cholesterol: 85 milligrams
Sodium: 685 milligrams
Potassium: 370 milligrams

Food Group Units:
Vegetables: 1½
Grains: 2
Meat and Alternatives:
        Moderately Low-Fat: 2

Stuffed Peppers

1 tablespoon vegetable oil
¾ cup chopped onion
½ cup chopped carrot
½ cup chopped celery
1 garlic clove, minced
2¼ cups low-sodium beef
   broth
½ teaspoon oregano, crushed
¼ teaspoon basil, crushed
¼ teaspoon salt
⅛ teaspoon pepper

81

1 cup barley
6 green peppers (about 2¼
    pounds)
½ cup tomato sauce
1½ ounces shredded
    part-skim mozzarella
    cheese (6 tablespoons)

In medium saucepan over medium-high heat in hot oil, cook onion, carrots, celery, and garlic about 5 minutes, stirring occasionally. Add beef broth, oregano, basil, salt, and pepper; bring to a boil. Add barley; reduce heat. Cover; simmer about 1 hour or until barley is tender, stirring occasionally.

Meanwhile, remove tops and seeds from peppers.

In large saucepan in 1-inch boiling water, heat peppers to boiling. Reduce heat to low; cover. Simmer about 5–7 minutes or until tender crisp.

Preheat oven to 375°F. In 1½-quart shallow baking dish, arrange peppers.

Stir tomato sauce into barley mixture.

Spoon an equal amount of filling into each pepper, approximately ¾ cup. Sprinkle with cheese. Cover and bake about 20–25 minutes. Makes 6 servings.

Approximate Nutrient Analysis Per Serving:
Calories: 215
Protein: 7 grams
Fat: 5 grams
Carbohydrate: 39 grams
Cholesterol: 4 milligrams
Sodium: 260 milligrams
Potassium: 560 milligrams

Food Group Units:
Vegetables: 2½
Grains: 1
Meat and Alternatives:
    Moderately Low-Fat: ½
Fat:
    Polyunsaturated: ½

Tuna Pasta Bake

2 teaspoons vegetable oil
½ cup chopped onion
1 garlic clove, minced
1 8-ounce can tomato sauce
½ teaspoon oregano
4 ounces spaghetti (2 cups
  cooked)
1 7-ounce can tuna in water,
  drained and flaked
½ cup cooked peas
1 cup low-fat cottage cheese
1 egg, slightly beaten
¼ teaspoon pepper
1½ tablespoons wheat germ

In small saucepan over medium-high heat in hot oil, cook onion and garlic, about 3 minutes, stirring occasionally. Add tomato sauce and oregano; bring to a boil. Reduce heat; cover. Simmer about 15 minutes, stirring occasionally.

Meanwhile, cook spaghetti as label directs, omitting salt. Drain; place in medium bowl. Add tuna and peas; toss well.

Preheat oven to 375°F.

In small bowl combine cottage cheese, egg, and pepper. Pour over spaghetti; mix well. In 1½-quart baking dish sprayed with non-stick cooking spray, place mixture. Pour sauce over mixture. Sprinkle with wheat germ. Bake 30 minutes until hot and bubbly. Makes 4 servings.

Approximate Nutrient Analysis Per Serving:
Calories: 285
Protein: 26 grams
Fat: 6 grams
Carbohydrate: 33 grams
Cholesterol: 95 milligrams
Sodium: 740 milligrams
Potassium: 550 milligrams

Food Group Units:
Vegetables: 2
Grains: 1½
Meat and Alternatives:

Very Low-Fat: 3

Fat:

Polyunsaturated: ½

Three Bean Bake

2 tablespoons vegetable oil,
    divided
¼ cup chopped onion
1 garlic clove, minced
1 16-ounce can white kidney
    beans, drained
1 16-ounce can chick peas,
    drained
1 16-ounce can tomatoes in
    juice, drained and chopped
1 8¾-ounce can red kidney
    beans, drained
2 teaspoons chili powder
⅛ teaspoon pepper
¾ cup cornmeal
¼ teaspoon baking soda
⅓ cup skim milk
1 egg, slightly beaten

In medium saucepan over medium-high heat in 1 tablespoon hot oil, cook onion and garlic about 3 minutes, stirring
occasionally. Add white kidney beans, chick peas, tomatoes,
red kidney beans, chili powder, and pepper; cover. Simmer
about 10 minutes, stirring occasionally. Into 1½-quart baking
dish sprayed with non-stick cooking spray, pour mixture.

Preheat oven to 375°F.

In small bowl, combine cornmeal and baking soda. Stir in
milk, egg, and remaining oil; mix well. Spoon over top of
beans. Bake about 20–25 minutes until cornmeal mixture is
lightly browned. Makes 8 servings.

Approximate Nutrient Analysis Per Serving:
Calories: 235
Protein: 11 grams
Fat: 6 grams
Carbohydrate: 36 grams

Cholesterol: 35 milligrams
Sodium: 465 milligrams
Potassium: 520 milligrams

Food Group Units:
Vegetables: 1
Legumes: 1½
Fat:
    Polyunsaturated: 1

Kasha and Mushrooms

1 tablespoon margarine
½ cup chopped onion
¼ cup sliced celery
¼ pound mushrooms, sliced
    (1½ cups)
½ cup kasha (buckwheat
    groats)
1 egg white, slightly beaten
1 cup low-sodium chicken
    broth
½ teaspoon salt
¼ teaspoon rosemary,
    crushed
⅛ teaspoon pepper

In large non-stick skillet over medium-high heat in hot
margarine, cook onion and celery about 4 minutes, stirring
occasionally. Add mushrooms; cook about 5 minutes, stirring
frequently. Combine kasha and egg white; add to skillet;
cook about 2 minutes, stirring frequently. Add remaining
ingredients; bring to a boil. Reduce heat; cover. Simmer
about 15–20 minutes or until all liquid is absorbed. Makes 4
servings.

Approximate Nutrient Analysis Per Serving:
Calories: 95
Protein: 4 grams
Fat: 4 grams
Carbohydrate: 14 grams

Cholesterol: 0
Sodium: 330 milligrams
Potassium: 270 milligrams

Food Group Units:
Vegetables: ½
Grains: 1
Fat:
    Polyunsaturated: ½

Gnocchi with Tomato Sauce

1 teaspoon vegetable oil
¼ cup finely chopped onion
2 garlic cloves, minced
1 8-ounce can tomato sauce
½ teaspoon Italian seasoning,
    crushed
⅛ teaspoon pepper
4 ounces part-skim ricotta
    cheese (½ cup)
4 tablespoons all-purpose
    flour
3 tablespoons grated
    Parmesan cheese
1 teaspoon margarine, melted
1 egg, lightly beaten

In small saucepan over medium-high heat in hot oil, cook
onion and garlic about 3 minutes, stirring frequently. Add
tomato sauce, Italian seasoning and pepper; bring to a boil.
Reduce heat; cover. Simmer about 10 minutes; keep warm.

In medium bowl, combine remaining ingredients. In large
saucepan over high heat, heat 3 quarts water to boiling.
With a tablespoon, drop cheese mixture into water. Simmer
about 3 minutes or until gnocchi float. Remove with slotted
spoon and drain. Arrange on broiler pan. Broil gnocchi
4 inches from heat, about 2 minutes on each side or until
lightly browned. Serve with tomato sauce. Makes 4 servings.

Approximate Nutrient Analysis Per Serving:

86

Calories: 150
Protein: 8 grams
Fat: 7 grams
Carbohydrate: 14 grams
Cholesterol: 80 milligrams
Sodium: 435 milligrams
Potassium: 305 milligrams

Food Group Units:
Vegetables: ½
Grains: ½
Meat and Alternatives:
    Moderately Low-Fat: 1
Fat:
    Saturated: ½

Eggplant Lasagna

1 medium eggplant, cut into
  very thin slices (1½ pounds)
1 tablespoon vegetable oil
½ cup chopped onion
1 pound mushrooms, sliced
9 lasagna noodles
1 15½-ounce jar spaghetti
  sauce
8 ounces part-skim ricotta
  cheese (1 cup)
4 ounces shredded part-skim
  mozzarella cheese (1 cup)
3 tablespoons grated
  Parmesan cheese

In large non-stick skillet sprayed with non-stick cooking spray, brown eggplant slices; set aside. In same skillet in hot oil, cook onion about 3 minutes, stirring occasionally. Add mushrooms; cook about 5–7 minutes or until mushrooms are tender, stirring frequently.

Cook lasagna noodles as label directs, omitting salt.

Preheat oven to 350°F.

In 11 x 7–inch baking dish, spoon ¼ cup of the sauce. Arrange three alternate layers of noodles, ricotta, mushroom mixture, mozzarella cheese, eggplant slices, sauce, and Parmesan cheese. Cover and bake about 30–40 minutes until heated through. Makes 8 servings.

Approximate Nutrient Analysis Per Serving:
Calories: 290
Protein: 15 grams
Fat: 11 grams
Carbohydrate: 36 grams
Cholesterol: 45 milligrams
Sodium: 400 milligrams
Potassium: 520 milligrams

Food Group Units:
Vegetables: 2
Grains: 1
Meat and Alternatives:
    Moderately Low-Fat: 2

Whole Wheat Pancakes with Rosy Applesauce

4 small red apples, cored and
    sliced
water
2 tablespoons sugar
1 teaspoon fresh lemon juice
⅛ teaspoon ground cinnamon
Dash ground cloves
⅓ cup whole wheat flour
⅓ cup all-purpose flour
1¼ teaspoons baking powder
½ cup milk
1 egg, slightly beaten
2 teaspoons vegetable oil
1½ teaspoons vanilla extract

In medium saucepan over low heat, combine apples, 3 tablespoons water, sugar, lemon juice, cinnamon, and cloves; bring to a boil. Reduce heat; cover. Simmer about 7–10 minutes or until apples are tender. Push mixture through a strainer into bowl. Cover and refrigerate until ready to use.

Preheat a non-stick griddle or griddle sprayed with non-stick cooking spray.

In small bowl, combine flours and baking powder. Stir in remaining ingredients and 3 tablespoons water until flour is moistened. Spoon 2 tablespoons of batter per pancake onto hot griddle; cook until golden brown on both sides. Serve with warm or chilled applesauce. Makes 5 servings, 2 pancakes each.

Approximate Nutrient Analysis Per Serving:
Calories: 180
Protein: 4 grams
Fat: 4 grams
Carbohydrate: 31 grams
Cholesterol: 60 milligrams
Sodium: 130 milligrams
Potassium: 190 milligrams

Food Group Units:
Fruit: 1
Grains: 1½
Fat:
      Polyunsaturated: 1

Red Snapper Stew

1 tablespoon vegetable oil
1 cup sliced celery (2 medium
   stalks)
1 cup sliced carrot (2
   medium)
½ cup chopped onion
½ cup chopped green pepper
2 garlic cloves, minced
1 16-ounce can tomatoes in
   juice, chopped
1 cup low-sodium chicken
   broth
¼ cup dry white wine
½ teaspoon dill weed
1 bay leaf

89

¼ teaspoon salt
¼ teaspoon pepper
1½ pounds red snapper
  fillets, cut into 1-inch
  pieces
½ cup water

In medium saucepan over medium-high heat in hot oil, cook celery, carrot, onion, green pepper, and garlic about 10 minutes or until tender-crisp, stirring occasionally. Add tomatoes in juice, chicken broth, wine, dill, bay leaf, salt, and pepper; bring to a boil. Reduce heat; cover. Simmer about 20 minutes. Add fish and water; bring to a boil. Reduce heat; simmer about 10 minutes or until fish flakes. Remove and discard bay leaf. Makes 6 servings, about 1 cup each.

Approximate Nutrient Analysis Per Serving:
Calories: 170
Protein: 24 grams
Fat: 4 grams
Carbohydrate: 9 grams
Cholesterol: 60 milligrams
Sodium: 30 milligrams
Potassium: 750 milligrams

Food Group Units:
Vegetables: 2
Meat and Alternatives:
    Very Low-Fat: 3

Sole Florentine

1 10-ounce package fresh or
  frozen spinach
4 sole fillets (1 pound)
1½ tablespoons margarine
2 tablespoons chopped onion
2 tablespoons all-purpose
  flour
1 cup skim milk
¼ teaspoon salt

⅛ teaspoon pepper
Dash ground nutmeg
1½ teaspoons grated
  Parmesan cheese
⅛ teaspoon paprika

Preheat oven to 350°F.

Cook spinach as label directs, omitting salt.

In 8-inch square baking dish sprayed with non-stick cooking spray, arrange spinach. Arrange fillets in single layer over spinach.

In small saucepan over low heat, melt margarine. Add onion; cook about 3 minutes or until soft, stirring frequently. Add flour; cook about 1 minute, stirring frequently. Gradually add milk, salt, pepper, and nutmeg; cook until thickened and smooth, stirring constantly. Pour over fish. Sprinkle with cheese and paprika. Bake about 15 minutes or until fish flakes. Makes 4 servings.

Approximate Nutrient Analysis Per Serving:
Calories: 185
Protein: 24 grams
Fat: 6 grams
Carbohydrate: 9 grams
Cholesterol: 60 milligrams
Sodium: 360 milligrams
Potassium: 760 milligrams

Food Group Units:
Vegetables: 1
Meat and Alternatives:
    Very Low-Fat: 3
Milk Products:
    Very Low-Fat: ¼
Fat:
    Polyunsaturated: ½

Crumb-Topped Fillets

2 tablespoons margarine,
  melted

2 tablespoons minced onion
1 tablespoon fresh lemon
   juice
3 walnut halves, chopped
1 small garlic clove, minced
½ teaspoon Italian seasoning,
   crushed
⅛ teaspoon pepper
4 flounder fillets (1 pound)
½ teaspoon paprika
¼ cup fresh whole wheat
   bread crumbs (about 1 slice
   bread)
fresh parsley sprigs

In small bowl, combine margarine, onion, lemon juice, walnuts, garlic, Italian seasoning, and pepper; mix well. Spoon an equal amount of mixture over each fillet. Sprinkle with paprika; top with bread crumbs. On broiler rack sprayed with non-stick cooking spray, place fish. Broil 3 to 4 inches from heat about 5–7 minutes or until topping is lightly browned and fish flakes easily. Garnish with parsley. Makes 4 servings.

Approximate Nutrient Analysis Per Serving:
Calories: 162
Protein: 20 grams
Fat: 8 grams
Carbohydrate: 3 grams
Cholesterol: 55 milligrams
Sodium: 170 milligrams
Potassium: 430 milligrams

Food Group Units:
Meat and Alternatives:
     Very Low-Fat: 3
Fat:
     Polyunsaturated: 1

Fillets en Papillote

4 flounder fillets (1 pound)

1 cup chopped tomatoes
(2 medium)
¼ cup minced green pepper
2 tablespoons minced onion
2 garlic cloves, minced
¼ teaspoon grated lemon
peel
2 teaspoons fresh lemon juice
½ teaspoon basil, crushed
¼ teaspoon salt
⅛ teaspoon pepper
4 teaspoons margarine

Preheat oven to 350°F.

On each of 4 pieces of aluminum foil or parchment paper large enough to wrap 1 fillet, place 1 fillet. Sprinkle fillets with equal amounts of tomatoes, green pepper, onion, garlic, lemon juice, basil, salt, lemon peel and pepper. Top each fillet with 1 teaspoon margarine. Wrap and seal all edges; place on baking pan. Bake about 20 minutes or until fish flakes. Makes 4 servings, about 3 ounces fish each.

Approximate Nutrient Analysis Per Serving:
Calories: 140
Protein: 20 grams
Fat: 5 grams
Carbohydrate: 4 grams
Cholesterol: 55 milligrams
Sodium: 270 milligrams
Potassium: 560 milligrams

Food Group Units:
Vegetables: 1
Meat and Alternatives:
Very Low-Fat: 3

Cold Poached Salmon with Curry Sauce

½ cup dry white wine
⅓ cup water
1 bay leaf
4–5 whole peppercorns

4 salmon steaks (1 pound)
½ cup plain low-fat yogurt
2 teaspoons mayonnaise
1 tablespoon finely chopped
    green onion
¾ teaspoon curry powder
⅛ teaspoon ground cumin

In large skillet, combine wine, water, bay leaf, and pepper; heat to boiling. Add salmon; cover. Simmer about 5–7 minutes or until fish flakes, turning once. Transfer to platter. Cover and refrigerate about 2 hours.

In small bowl, combine remaining ingredients. Serve with salmon. Makes 4 servings, about 3 ounces salmon each.

Approximate Nutrient Analysis Per Serving:
Calories: 290
Protein: 27 grams
Fat: 18 grams
Carbohydrate: 4 grams
Cholesterol: 45 milligrams
Sodium: 120 milligrams
Potassium: 585 milligrams

Food Group Units:
Grains: ¼
Meat and Alternatives:
    Moderately Low-Fat: 3½
Fat:
    Polyunsaturated: ½

Sweet and Sour Fillets

1½ teaspoons vegetable oil
2 tablespoons chopped onion
2 tablespoons chopped red
    pepper
1 small garlic clove, minced
¼ cup + 1 tablespoon water
1 tablespoon red wine vinegar
1 tablespoon sugar

1½ teaspoons dry sherry
¾ teaspoon soy sauce
Dash pepper
4 flounder fillets, cut in half*
  (1 pound)
1 teaspoon cornstarch
chopped fresh parsley

In large non-stick skillet over medium-high heat in hot oil, cook onion, red pepper, and garlic about 4 minutes or until soft, stirring frequently. Add ½ cup water, vinegar, sugar, sherry, soy sauce, and pepper; heat to boiling. Add fillets; cover. Simmer about 10 minutes or until fish flakes easily. With slotted spatula, transfer fillets to serving platter; keep warm.

In small bowl, combine cornstarch and 2 tablespoons water; add to skillet. Cook about 1 minute or until thickened, stirring constantly. Pour over fillets. Sprinkle with parsley. Makes 4 servings, about 3 ounces fish each.

Approximate Nutrient Analysis Per Serving:
Calories: 125
Protein: 19 grams
Fat: 3 grams
Carbohydrate: 5 grams
Cholesterol: 55 milligrams
Sodium: 185 milligrams
Potassium: 415 milligrams

Food Group Units:
Grains: ⅓
Meat and Alternatives:
    Very Low-Fat: 3

*Thin chicken cutlets may be substituted for fish fillets; increase cooking time by about 10 minutes.

Salmon Loaf

1 15½-ounce can canned
    salmon, drained and flaked
    (2 cups)

1 cup fresh whole wheat
  bread crumbs (2 slices
  bread)
1 cup cooked rice
1 egg, slightly beaten
1 egg white, slightly beaten
¼ cup skim milk
2 tablespoons minced onion
1 tablespoon fresh lemon
  juice
½ teaspoon dill weed
⅛ teaspoon pepper

Preheat oven to 375°F.

In large bowl, combine all ingredients; mix well. Into 9 x 5–inch loaf pan sprayed with non-stick cooking spray, spoon mixture, pressing down mixture lightly. Bake about 45 minutes or until knife inserted in center comes out clean; invert onto serving platter. Makes 8 servings.

Approximate Nutrient Analysis Per Serving:
Calories: 135
Protein: 14 grams
Fat: 4 grams
Carbohydrate: 10 grams
Cholesterol: 55 milligrams
Sodium: 260 milligrams
Potassium: 255 milligrams

Food Group Units:
Grains: 1
Meat and Alternatives:
    Moderately Low-Fat: 1

Lemon-Bread Stuffed Fish

1 tablespoon margarine
¼ cup chopped onion
¼ cup chopped celery
1 garlic clove, minced
1½ cups fresh whole wheat

bread crumbs
2 tablespoons chopped fresh
  parsley
2 tablespoons fresh lemon
  juice, divided
1 tablespoon dry white wine
½ teaspoon grated lemon
  peel
¼ teaspoon thyme, crushed
¼ teaspoon salt
⅛ teaspoon pepper
1½ pounds pan-dressed fish
  (trout or striped bass), head
  and tail removed

Preheat oven to 350°F.
In medium saucepan over medium-high heat in hot margarine, cook onion, celery, and garlic about 4 minutes or until soft. Remove from heat; stir in bread crumbs, parsley, 1 tablespoon lemon juice, wine, lemon peel, thyme, salt, and pepper. Fill cavity of fish with stuffing, securing with toothpicks or skewers; place in baking dish sprayed with non-stick cooking spray or lined with aluminum foil. Sprinkle with remaining lemon juice; cover. Bake about 40 minutes or until fish flakes. Makes 4 servings.

Approximate Nutrient Analysis Per Serving:
Calories: 235
Protein: 32 grams
Fat: 7 grams
Carbohydrate: 11 grams
Cholesterol: 75 milligrams
Sodium: 340 milligrams
Potassium: 610 milligrams

Food Group Units:
Grains: 1
Meat and Alternatives:
    Very Low-Fat: 3½
Fat:
    Polyunsaturated: 1

Mexican Baked Fish

1 tablespoon vegetable oil
¼ cup chopped onion
2 garlic cloves, minced
1 16-ounce can tomatoes in
  juice, drained and chopped
1 tablespoon chopped green
  chilies
1 teaspoon chili powder
⅛ teaspoon pepper
1 egg white
1 tablespoon skim milk
½ cup cornmeal
4 flounder fillets (1 pound)
2 ounces shredded part-skim
  mozzarella cheese (½ cup)

Preheat oven to 350°F.

In small saucepan over medium-high heat in hot oil, cook onion and garlic about 3 minutes until soft, stirring frequently. Add tomatoes, chilies, chili powder, and pepper; bring to a boil. Reduce heat; cover. Simmer about 15 minutes, stirring occasionally.

In shallow dish, beat egg white and skim milk slightly. On waxed paper, place cornmeal. Dip fillets in egg mixture; coat in cornmeal. In baking dish sprayed with non-stick cooking spray, place fillets in single layer. Pour sauce over fish; sprinkle with cheese. Bake about 20 minutes or until fish flakes. Makes 4 servings, about 3 ounces fish each.

Approximate Nutrient Analysis Per Serving:
Calories: 255
Protein: 26 grams
Fat: 7 grams
Carbohydrate: 21 grams
Cholesterol: 65 milligrams
Sodium: 325 milligrams
Potassium: 720 milligrams

Food Group Units:
Vegetables: 1
Grains: 1
Meat and Alternatives:

Fat: Very Low-Fat: 3½

Polyunsaturated: 1

Chicken Enchiladas

1 tablespoon vegetable oil,
  divided
2 garlic cloves, minced
1 16-ounce can tomatoes in
  juice, chopped
1 tablespoon chili powder,
  divided
⅛ teaspoon pepper
1½ cups chopped cooked
  chicken (about 8 ounces
  cooked)
¼ cup plain low-fat yogurt
3 tablespoons chopped green
  chilies
2 tablespoons finely chopped
  green onion
4 corn tortillas
2 ounces shredded part-skim
  mozzarella cheese

In medium saucepan over medium heat in 2 teaspoons hot oil, cook garlic about 1 minute. Add tomatoes, 2 teaspoons chili powder, and pepper; simmer uncovered about 30 minutes, stirring occasionally.

Meanwhile, in small bowl combine chicken, yogurt, green chilies, green onion, and remaining chili powder; mix well.

In large non-stick skillet in remaining hot oil, add tortillas, one at a time. Cook about 1 minute on each side or until soft.

Meanwhile, preheat oven to 350°F.

Spoon ¼ cup sauce into 8-inch square baking dish. In center of each tortilla, spread an equal amount of chicken mixture. Fold sides over filling. In baking dish, over sauce, place tortilla seam-side down. Pour sauce over tortillas. Sprinkle with cheese. Bake about 30 minutes or until heated through. Makes 4 servings.

Approximate Nutrient Analysis Per Serving:
Calories: 260
Protein: 23 grams
Fat: 11 grams
Carbohydrate: 18 grams
Cholesterol: 60 milligrams
Sodium: 290 milligrams
Potassium: 480 milligrams

Food Group Units:
Vegetables: 1
Grains: 1
Meat and Alternatives:
    Very Low-Fat: 2½
    Moderately Low-Fat: ½
Fat:
    Polyunsaturated: 1

Chicken Bundles

2 whole chicken breasts, split,
  skinned, and boned
  (1 pound boneless)
1 tablespoon margarine,
  divided
2 tablespoons finely chopped
  onion
1 cup mashed sweet potatoes
  (about 2 potatoes)
2 tablespoons dry white wine
2 teaspoons honey
½ teaspoon grated orange
  peel
¼ teaspoon salt
⅛ teaspoon ground cinnamon
Dash ground nutmeg
Dash pepper
2 tablespoons natural barley
  cereal

100

Preheat oven to 400°F.

On cutting board with meat mallet, pound chicken to ¼-inch thickness; set aside.

In small skillet over medium heat in 1 teaspoon hot margarine, cook onion about 3 minutes or until soft. Stir in sweet potato, wine, honey, orange peel, salt, cinnamon, nutmeg, and pepper; cook about 1 minute.

With a tablespoon, spoon mixture onto each chicken breast; roll up and secure with toothpicks. In 8-inch square baking dish, place roll-ups seam-side down. Cover; bake about 20 minutes or until chicken is tender.

Meanwhile, in small saucepan over medium heat, melt remaining margarine.

Sprinkle bundles with cereal; drizzle melted margarine over top. Increase oven heat to broil. Broil chicken about 3–4 inches from heat about 1 minute or until lightly browned. Makes 4 servings, about 3 ounces chicken each.

Approximate Nutrient Analysis Per Serving:
Calories: 250
Protein: 28 grams
Fat: 5 grams
Carbohydrate: 23 grams
Cholesterol: 65 milligrams
Sodium: 275 milligrams

Food Group Units:
Vegetables: 1
Grains: 1
Meat and Alternatives:
    Very Low-Fat: 3
Fat:
    Polyunsaturated: ½

Chicken and Rice Skillet

2 whole chicken breasts, split,
    skinned and boned
    (1 pound boneless), cut
    into bite-size pieces
¼ teaspoon salt
⅛ teaspoon pepper

101

1 16-ounce can tomatoes in
  juice, chopped
½ cup water
½ cup chopped onion
¼ cup chopped green pepper
2 garlic cloves, minced
½ teaspoon oregano, crushed
½ cup long-grain rice

Season chicken with salt and pepper. In large non-stick
skillet or skillet sprayed with non-stick cooking spray over
medium-high heat, brown chicken. Add tomatoes in juice,
water, onion, green pepper, garlic, and oregano; bring to a
boil.

Stir in rice; return to a boil. Reduce heat; cover. Simmer
about 20–25 minutes or until liquid is absorbed and chicken is
tender, stirring occasionally, turning chicken once. Makes 4
servings, about 3 ounces chicken each.

Approximate Nutrient Analysis Per Serving:
Calories: 250
Protein: 29 grams
Fat: 2 grams
Carbohydrate: 26 grams
Cholesterol: 65 milligrams
Sodium: 360 milligrams
Potassium: 604 milligrams

Food Group Units:
Vegetables: 1½
Grains: 1
Meat and Alternatives:
    Very Low-Fat: 3

Chicken and Vegetables Stir Fry

⅓ cup low-sodium chicken
  broth
2 tablespoons dry sherry
1 tablespoon low-sodium soy
  sauce
1 tablespoon cornstarch

⅛ teaspoon pepper
2 whole chicken breasts, split,
   skinned and boned
   (1 pound boneless), cut
   into ½-inch pieces
1 tablespoon peanut oil
1 6-ounce package frozen
   snow peas, thawed and
   well drained
¼ pound mushrooms, sliced
   (1½ cups)
2 tablespoons chopped green
   onion
2 garlic cloves, minced
¼ teaspoon finely chopped
   ginger root

In shallow dish, combine chicken broth, sherry, soy sauce, cornstarch, and pepper. Add chicken; toss well. Cover and refrigerate about 1 hour, stirring occasionally.

In large non-stick skillet over high heat in hot oil, add snow peas, mushrooms, green onion, garlic, and ginger root; cook about 3–5 minutes or until tender-crisp. Remove from skillet; set aside.

Add chicken with marinade to skillet; cook about 10 minutes or until chicken is tender and sauce is thickened, stirring occasionally. If necessary, add about ¼ cup water to skillet.

Return vegetables to skillet; cook about 1 minute, stirring frequently. Makes 4 servings, about ¾ cup each.

Approximate Nutrient Analysis Per Serving:
Calories: 210
Protein: 29 grams
Fat: 6 grams
Carbohydrate: 10 grams
Cholesterol: 65 milligrams
Sodium: 130 milligrams
Potassium: 495 milligrams

Food Group Units:
Vegetables: 2
Meat and Alternatives:
    Very Low-Fat: 3

Fat:
  Monounsaturated: 1

Orange Chicken

1 tablespoon vegetable oil
2 whole chicken breasts, split,
    skinned and boned
    (1 pound boneless)
1 cup red pepper, cut into
    chunks (1 medium)
2 tablespoons chopped green
    onion
1 garlic clove, minced
¾ cup orange juice
1 teaspoon prepared mustard
¼ teaspoon salt
⅛ teaspoon pepper
2 teaspoons cornstarch
2 tablespoons water
½ cup fresh orange sections,
    cut into bite-size pieces
    (½ medium)

In large non-stick skillet over medium-high heat in hot oil, brown chicken. Remove from skillet.

Add red pepper, green onion, and garlic; cook about 5 minutes or until tender, stirring occasionally.

Return chicken to skillet. Add orange juice, mustard, salt, and pepper; bring to a boil. Reduce heat; cover. Simmer about 20 minutes. Transfer chicken to serving platter; keep warm.

In small bowl, combine cornstarch and water; add to skillet. Increase heat to high heat; add orange sections. Cook about 1–2 minutes or until thickened, stirring frequently. Pour over chicken. Garnish with parsley. Makes 4 servings, about 3 ounces chicken each.

Approximate Nutrient Analysis Per Serving:
Calories: 210
Protein: 28 grams
Fat: 6 grams

Carbohydrate: 12 grams
Cholesterol: 65 milligrams
Sodium: 235 milligrams
Potassium: 495 milligrams

Food Group Units:
Vegetables: 2
Fruit: 1
Meat and Alternatives:
    Very Low-Fat: 3

Chicken Divan

4 whole chicken breasts, split,
  skinned and boned
  (1 pound boneless, raw)
1 10-ounce package frozen
  broccoli spears, cooked
  and drained (or 2 cups
  fresh, steamed)
2 tablespoons margarine
¼ cup chopped onion
¼ cup all-purpose flour
1½ cups skim milk
2 tablespoons dry sherry
⅛ teaspoon salt
⅛ teaspoon pepper
Dash ground nutmeg
1½ tablespoons grated
  Parmesan cheese

Preheat oven to 400°F.
In non-stick skillet sprayed with non-stick cooking spray
over medium-high heat, brown chicken breasts.
In 8-inch square baking pan, arrange broccoli. Place chick-
en in single layer over broccoli.
In medium saucepan, over low heat, or in double boiler,
melt margarine. Add onion; cook about 3 minutes, stirring
frequently. Stir in flour; cook about 1 minute, stirring constantly. Gradually add milk, sherry, salt, pepper, and nutmeg; cook until thickened and smooth, stirring constantly.
Pour over chicken and broccoli. Sprinkle with cheese. Bake

about 20 minutes or until bubbly. Makes 4 servings, about 3 ounces chicken each.

Approximate Nutrient Analysis Per Serving:
Calories: 280
Protein: 34 grams
Fat: 9 grams
Carbohydrate: 17 grams
Cholesterol: 70 milligrams
Sodium: 355 milligrams
Potassium: 732 milligrams

Food Group Units:
Vegetables: 1
Grains: ½
Meat and Alternatives:
    Very Low-Fat: 3
Milk Products:
    Very Low-Fat: ½
Fat:
    Polyunsaturated: 1

Chicken with Currant Sauce

2 whole chicken breasts, split,
    skinned, and boned
    (1 pound boneless)
1 tablespoon margarine
2 tablespoons finely chopped
    onion
1 garlic clove, minced
½ cup currant jelly
¼ cup raisins
⅛ teaspoon dry mustard
⅛ teaspoon salt
⅛ teaspoon pepper
2 teaspoons cornstarch
2 tablespoons water

Preheat oven to 400°F.
In 8-inch square baking dish sprayed with non-stick cook-

106

ing spray, place chicken. Cover; bake about 20–30 minutes or until tender.

Meanwhile, in small saucepan over medium heat in hot margarine, cook onion and garlic about 3 minutes or until soft. Add jelly, raisins, mustard, salt, and pepper; cook until jelly is melted, stirring constantly.

In small bowl, combine cornstarch and water; mix well. Add to saucepan; cook until thickened, stirring constantly. Serve sauce with chicken. Makes 4 servings, about 3 ounces chicken each.

Approximate Nutrient Analysis Per Serving:
Calories: 295
Protein: 27 grams
Fat: 5 grams
Carbohydrate: 36 grams
Cholesterol: 65 milligrams
Sodium: 190 milligrams
Potassium: 380 milligrams

Food Group Units:
Fruit: 1
Grains: 1½
Meat and Alternatives:
    Very Low-Fat: 3
Fat:
    Polyunsaturated: 1

Chicken with Wine Sauce

1 tablespoon vegetable oil
2 whole chicken breasts, split,
    skinned, and boned
    (1 pound boneless)
½ pound mushrooms, sliced
    (3½ cups)
¼ cup chopped onion
2 garlic cloves, minced
½ cup dry red wine
⅓ cup + 1½ tablespoons
    water

107

¼ teaspoon thyme, crushed
¼ teaspoon salt
⅛ teaspoon pepper
2 teaspoons all-purpose flour
2 tablespoons chopped fresh
  parsley

In large non-stick skillet over medium heat in hot oil, brown chicken. Remove from skillet.

Add mushrooms, onion, and garlic to drippings in skillet; cook about 5 minutes or until tender, stirring occasionally. Return chicken to skillet. Add red wine, ⅓ cup water, thyme, salt, and pepper; bring to a boil. Reduce heat; cover. Simmer about 20 minutes or until chicken is tender, turning once. Transfer chicken to serving platter; keep warm.

In small bowl, combine flour and 1½ tablespoons water; add to skillet. Cook about 1 minute, stirring constantly. Stir in parsley. Spoon sauce over chicken. Makes 4 servings.

Approximate Nutrient Analysis Per Serving:
Calories: 195
Protein: 28 grams
Fat: 6 grams
Carbohydrate: 6 grams
Cholesterol: 65 milligrams
Sodium: 225 milligrams
Potassium: 575 milligrams

Food Group Units:
Vegetables: 1
Meat and Alternatives:
    Very Low-Fat: 3
Fat:
    Polyunsaturated: 1

Spicy Chicken Wings

2 pounds chicken wings,
  halved and skinned (about
  12–16)

¾ cup plain low-fat yogurt
1 tablespoon vegetable oil
1 tablespoon dry sherry
1 garlic clove, minced
½ teaspoon finely chopped
   ginger root
½ teaspoon grated orange
   peel
⅛ teaspoon ground red
   pepper
1½ cups crushed unsalted,
   whole-grain crackers
   (about 36)
¼ cup toasted sesame seeds

In shallow dish, place chicken wings.

In small bowl, combine yogurt, oil, sherry, garlic, ginger root, orange peel, and red pepper. Pour over wings; toss well. Cover and refrigerate about 2 hours, stirring occasionally.

Preheat oven to 375°F.

In shallow dish, combine cracker crumbs and sesame seeds. Coat chicken wings evenly with crumb mixture; place on baking pan sprayed with non-stick cooking spray. Bake about 30 minutes. Makes 4 servings.

Approximate Nutrient Analysis Per Serving:
Calories: 340
Protein: 27 grams
Fat: 16 grams
Carbohydrate: 23 grams
Cholesterol: 60 milligrams
Sodium: 340 milligrams
Potassium: 360 milligrams

Food Group Units:
Grains: 1½
Meat and Alternatives:
     Very Low-Fat: 3
Fat:
     Polyunsaturated: 2½

2 10-ounce packages frozen
  lima beans
1½ cups cooked, cubed
  chicken (9 ounces cooked)
1 16-ounce can tomatoes in
  juice, drained and chopped
¼ cup finely chopped onion
1 clove garlic, minced
4 ounces shredded part-skim
  mozzarella cheese (1 cup)
1½ teaspoons dry mustard
1 teaspoon Worcestershire
  sauce
⅛ teaspoon pepper
¼ cup fresh whole wheat
  bread crumbs

Preheat oven to 375°F.
Prepare beans as label directs, omitting salt.
In 1½-quart baking dish sprayed with non-stick cooking spray, place beans.
In large bowl, combine chicken, tomatoes, onion, garlic, mustard, Worcestershire sauce, and pepper; mix well. Pour mixture over top of beans. Sprinkle cheese and bread-crumbs over bean mixture. Bake about 30 minutes or until hot and bubbly. Makes 6 servings.

Approximate Nutrient Analysis Per Serving:
Calories: 250
Protein: 24 grams
Fat: 7 grams
Carbohydrate: 24 grams
Cholesterol: 50 milligrams
Sodium: 365 milligrams
Potassium: 770 milligrams

Food Group Units:
Vegetables: 1
Legumes: 1
Meat and Alternatives:
    Very Low-Fat: 2½

Fat:
Saturated: ½

Turkey Tetrazzini

4 ounces spaghetti (2 cups
  cooked)
1 tablespoon margarine
¼ pound mushrooms, sliced
  (1½ cups)
2 tablespoons chopped onion
2 tablespoons all-purpose
  flour
1½ cups skim milk
1 tablespoon dry sherry
¼ teaspoon salt
⅛ teaspoon pepper
⅛ teaspoon ground nutmeg
1½ cups cooked, cubed
  turkey or chicken
  (9 ounces cooked)
2 tablespoons chopped
  pimento
3 tablespoons grated
  Parmesan cheese

Preheat oven to 350°F.

Cook spaghetti as label directs, omitting salt.

Meanwhile, in small saucepan over medium-high heat in margarine, cook mushrooms and onion about 4 minutes, stirring occasionally. Add flour; cook about 1 minute, stirring constantly. Gradually add milk, sherry, salt, pepper, and nutmeg; cook about 5 minutes or until thickened, stirring constantly.

In 1-quart casserole dish sprayed with non-stick cooking spray, place spaghetti, turkey, pimento, and sauce; toss well. Sprinkle with cheese, cover. Bake 20–25 minutes or until hot and bubbly. Makes 4 servings.

Approximate Nutrient Analysis Per Serving:
Calories: 315
Protein: 28 grams

Fat: 8 grams
Carbohydrate: 32 grams
Cholesterol: 55 milligrams
Sodium: 365 milligrams
Potassium: 555 milligrams

Food Group Units:
Vegetables: 1
Grains: 1½
Meat and Alternatives:
    Very Low-Fat: 2½
Milk Products:
    Very Low-Fat: ½
Fat:
    Polyunsaturated: 1

Veal Stew

1½ pounds veal stew meat,
  cut into 1-inch pieces
2 tablespoons all-purpose
  flour
2 tablespoons margarine
2 small onions, peeled and
  cut into quarters
1 garlic clove, minced
1½ cup low-sodium beef
  broth
½ cup dry white wine
1 bay leaf
½ teaspoon thyme, crushed
½ teaspoon salt
⅛ teaspoon pepper
4 carrots, peeled and cut in
  chunks
2 small potatoes, peeled and
  cut in chunks
½ cup water

In plastic bag, combine flour and meat; toss to coat.

In a large saucepan over medium-high heat in hot margarine, brown veal. Reduce heat to medium; add onions and

garlic to drippings in saucepan. Cook about 5 minutes or until soft, stirring occasionally.

Add beef broth, wine, bay leaf, thyme, salt, and pepper; bring to a boil. Reduce heat; cover. Simmer about 1¼ hours. Add carrots, potatoes, and water; continue to simmer about 45 minutes or until meat and vegetables are tender.

Remove cover; cook additional 10 minutes over medium-high heat. Remove and discard bay leaf. Makes 6 servings, about 1 cup each.

Approximate Nutrient Analysis Per Serving:
Calories: 305
Protein: 24 grams
Fat: 16 grams
Carbohydrate: 17 grams
Cholesterol: 80 milligrams
Sodium: 330 milligrams
Potassium: 757 milligrams

Food Group Units:
Vegetables: 2
Grains: ½
Meat and Alternatives:
    Moderately Low-Fat: 3

Veal Chops with Mushrooms

4 veal rib chops, about
    ¾-inch thick (2 pounds)
¼ teaspoon salt
1 tablespoon margarine
¼ cup chopped onion
1 garlic clove, minced
½ pound mushrooms, sliced
    (3 cups)
1 16-ounce can tomatoes in
    juice, chopped
2 tablespoons dry red wine
¼ teaspoon rosemary,
    crushed
⅛ teaspoon pepper

113

Trim fat from chops and season with salt. In large non-stick skillet sprayed with non-stick cooking spray over medium-high heat, brown veal chops. Remove from skillet.

Add margarine, onion, and garlic to skillet; cook about 3 minutes or until soft, stirring occasionally. Add mushrooms; cook about 5 minutes, stirring occasionally. Add tomatoes in juice, wine, salt, rosemary, and pepper; bring to a boil. Reduce heat; return chops to skillet. Cover, simmer about 45 minutes or until veal is tender, turning occasionally. Transfer chops to serving platter; keep warm.

Increase heat to high; cook sauce, about 5–7 minutes or until reduced and slightly thickened, stirring frequently. Spoon sauce over chops. Makes 4 servings, about 8 ounces of veal each.

Approximate Nutrient Analysis Per Serving:
Calories: 395
Protein: 36 grams
Fat: 24 grams
Carbohydrate: 9 grams
Cholesterol: 120 milligrams
Sodium: 405 milligrams
Potassium: 875 milligrams

Food Group Units:
Vegetables: 2
Meat and Alternatives:
    Moderately Low-Fat: 4
Fat:
    Polyunsaturated: 1

Veal Piccata

4 veal cutlets, about ¼-inch
   thick (1 pound)
2 tablespoons all-purpose
   flour
2 teaspoons margarine
1 teaspoon olive oil
1 garlic clove, minced
¼ cup chopped fresh parsley

114

1 tablespoon fresh lemon
  juice
⅛ teaspoon grated lemon
  peel
¼ teaspoon salt
⅛ teaspoon pepper
2 tablespoons water

On cutting board with meat mallet, pound veal cutlets to ⅛-inch thickness. Coat with flour, shaking off excess.

In large non-stick skillet over medium-high heat in hot margarine and oil, brown cutlets. Remove from skillet.

Add remaining ingredients, except water, to skillet; cook about 2 minutes, stirring frequently. Return veal to skillet; add water. Reduce heat; cover. Simmer about 10–15 minutes or until veal is tender. Makes 4 servings.

Approximate Nutrient Analysis Per Serving:
Calories: 230
Protein: 23 grams
Fat: 13 grams
Carbohydrate: 4 grams
Cholesterol: 80 milligrams
Sodium: 235 milligrams
Potassium: 400 milligrams

Food Group Units:
Vegetables: 1
Meat and Alternatives:
    Moderately Low-Fat: 3

Stuffed Veal Rolls

4 veal cutlets, about ¼-inch
  thick (1 pound)
1 tablespoon margarine
¼ cup finely chopped celery
2 tablespoons finely chopped
  onion
1 garlic clove, minced
1 cup fresh whole wheat

115

bread crumbs (about 2 slices)
1 tablespoon chopped fresh
    parsley
¼ teaspoon salt
¼ teaspoon sage
¼ teaspoon pepper
1 cup low-sodium beef broth
¼ pound mushrooms, sliced
    (about ½ cup)
2 teaspoons flour
2 tablespoons water

On cutting board with meat mallet, pound veal cutlets to
⅛-inch thickness; set aside.

In small saucepan over medium-high heat in hot margarine,
cook celery, onion, and garlic about 5 minutes until tender,
stirring occasionally. Remove from heat; stir in bread
crumbs, parsley, and seasonings.

With tablespoon, spoon stuffing onto each veal cutlet; roll
up and secure with toothpicks.

In large non-stick skillet sprayed with non-stick cooking
spray, over medium heat, brown veal rolls on all sides. Add
beef broth and mushrooms; bring to a boil. Reduce heat;
cover. Simmer about 20–30 minutes or until veal is fork
tender. Transfer veal to serving platter; keep warm.

In small bowl, combine flour and water; mix well. Add to
liquid in skillet; cook until thickened, stirring constantly. Pour over veal. Makes 4 servings, about 3 ounces veal
each.

Approximate Nutrient Analysis Per Serving:
Calories: 262
Protein: 25 grams
Fat: 14 grams
Carbohydrate: 10 grams
Cholesterol: 80 milligrams
Sodium: 320 milligrams
Potassium: 580 milligrams

Food Group Units:
Vegetables: ½
Grains: ½
Meat and Alternatives:
    Moderately Low-Fat: 3

Veal Loaf

1¼ pounds ground veal
¼ pound ground pork
1 cup fresh whole wheat
   bread crumbs (about 2
   slices)
½ cup chopped onion
   (1 small)
¼ cup chopped green pepper
   (½ small)
¼ cup chopped celery
   (1 medium stalk)
2 garlic cloves, minced
1 egg, slightly beaten
¼ cup skim milk
¼ cup chopped fresh parsley
¼ teaspoon thyme, crushed
¼ teaspoon dill weed
¼ teaspoon grated lemon
   peel
¼ teaspoon salt
⅛ teaspoon pepper

Preheat oven to 375°F.

In a large bowl, combine all ingredients; mix well. Spoon into a 9 x 5-inch loaf pan sprayed with non-stick cooking spray; level top. Bake about 1–1¼ hours or until lightly browned and loaf pulls slightly away from side of pan. Let stand about 10 minutes before inverting onto platter. Makes 6 servings, about 1¾ inches thick each.

Approximate Nutrient Analysis Per Serving:
Calories:　235
Protein:　23 grams
Fat:　13 grams
Carbohydrate:　7 grams
Cholesterol:　120 milligrams
Sodium:　195 milligrams
Potassium:　300 milligrams

Food Group Units:
Grains:　½

Veal Parmigiana

4 veal cutlets, about ¼-inch
    thick (1 pound)
½ cup plain dry bread crumbs
2¼ teaspoons grated
    Parmesan cheese
1 egg
1 tablespoon water
1 tablespoon olive oil
1½ cups no-added-salt
    spaghetti sauce
½ cup shredded part-skim
    mozzarella cheese
    (2 ounces)
¼ teaspoon oregano, crushed

Preheat oven to 375°F.

On cutting board with meat mallet, pound veal cutlets to
⅛-inch thickness.

In shallow dish, combine bread crumbs and Parmesan
cheese; mix well.

In another shallow dish, beat egg and water slightly. Dip
veal into egg mixture, then coat with bread crumb mixture.

In large non-stick skillet over medium-high heat in hot oil,
brown veal.

In a shallow 2-quart baking dish, arrange cutlets in a single
layer. Pour sauce over veal. Sprinkle with mozzarella cheese
and oregano. Bake about 20–30 minutes or until bubbly.
Makes 4 servings, about 4 ounces veal each.

Approximate Nutrient Analysis Per Serving:
Calories: 385
Protein: 30 grams
Fat: 21 grams
Carbohydrate: 17 grams
Cholesterol: 160 milligrams
Sodium: 305 milligrams
Potassium: 405 milligrams

Food Group Units:
Vegetables: 1
Meat and Alternatives:
    Moderately Low-Fat: 4
Fat:
    Monounsaturated: 1

Veal and Peppers

4 veal cutlets, about ¼-inch
   thick (1 pound)
1½ tablespoons olive oil
1½ cups green pepper strips
   (1 large)
1½ cups red pepper strips
   (1 large)
½ cup sliced onion
2 garlic cloves, minced
¼ cup dry white wine
¼ teaspoon salt
¼ teaspoon sage leaves
⅛ teaspoon pepper

On cutting board with meat mallet, pound veal cutlets to ⅛-inch thickness. Cut into ½-inch strips. In large non-stick skillet over medium-high heat in hot oil, brown veal. Remove from skillet.

Reduce heat to medium; add red and green peppers, onion, and garlic. Cook about 7 minutes or until soft, stirring occasionally.

Return veal to skillet; add remaining ingredients. Cook about 15–20 minutes or until tender, stirring occasionally. If necessary add about 1–2 tablespoons water. Makes 4 servings, about 4 ounces veal each.

Approximate Nutrient Analysis Per Serving:
Calories: 275
Protein: 25 grams
Fat: 16 grams
Carbohydrate: 10 grams
Cholesterol: 80 milligrams

Sodium: 230 milligrams
Potassium: 650 milligrams

Food Group Units:
Vegetables: 2
Meat and Alternatives:
        Moderately Low-Fat: 3

Moussaka

1½–1¾ pounds eggplant,
    peeled and sliced ¼ inch
    thick (1½ medium)
1 pound ground lamb,
    trimmed of visible fat
    before grinding
½ cup chopped onion
2 garlic cloves, minced
½ cup tomato sauce
¼ cup dry red wine
½ teaspoon oregano, crushed
¼ teaspoon salt, divided
¼ teaspoon pepper, divided
¼ teaspoon ground cinnamon
3 tablespoons all-purpose
    flour, divided
2 tablespoons water
1 tablespoon margarine
1½ cups skim milk
1 tablespoon grated Parmesan
    cheese

In large non-stick skillet sprayed with non-stick cooking
spray, brown eggplant slices; set aside. In same skillet, brown
lamb. Drain and discard excess fat. Add onion and garlic to
skillet; cook about 3 minutes, stirring frequently. Add tomato
sauce, wine, oregano, ⅛ teaspoon salt, ⅛ teaspoon pepper
and cinnamon; cook about 20 minutes, stirring occasionally.

In small bowl, combine 1 tablespoon flour and water. Add
to skillet; cook about 2 minutes, stirring constantly. Remove
from heat.

Preheat oven to 325°F.

In 11 x 7–inch baking pan sprayed with non-stick cooking spray, layer half of the eggplant slices. Cover with lamb mixture. Top with remaining eggplant slices.

In small saucepan over low heat, melt margarine. Add remaining flour; cook about 1 minute, stirring constantly. Gradually add milk and remaining salt and pepper; cook about 7–10 minutes or until thickened, stirring constantly. Pour sauce over eggplant slices. Sprinkle with cheese. Bake about 30–40 minutes or until hot and bubbly. Makes 6 servings.

Approximate Nutrient Analysis Per Serving:
Calories: 280
Protein: 16 grams
Fat: 17 grams
Carbohydrate: 17 grams
Cholesterol: 55 milligrams
Sodium: 290 milligrams
Potassium: 610 milligrams

Food Group Units:
Vegetables: 2
Grains: ½
Meat and Alternatives:
    Moderately Low-Fat: 2
Fat:
    Polyunsaturated: 1

Lamb Shish Kabobs

3 tablespoons fresh lemon
    juice
1 tablespoon olive oil
2 small garlic cloves, minced
¾ teaspoon oregano, crushed
⅛ teaspoon pepper
1 pound boneless lamb, cut
    into 16 cubes
1 large green pepper, cut into
    16 squares (about 1½ cups)

2 onions, each cut into 8
   wedges (2 cups)
1 cup plain low-fat yogurt

In shallow dish, combine lemon juice, oil, garlic, oregano, and pepper. Add lamb; toss well. Cover and refrigerate about 1 hour, stirring occasionally.

Remove lamb from marinade, reserving marinade. On each of four skewers, arrange 4 pieces of lamb, 4 green pepper squares, and 4 onion wedges, then place on broiler pan lined with foil. Broil 4 inches from heat about 30–35 minutes, turning often and brushing with reserved marinade. Transfer kabobs to serving platter.

In small bowl, place yogurt. Pour drippings from broiler pan into yogurt and mix well. Serve with kabobs. Makes 4 servings.

Approximate Nutrient Analysis Per Serving:
Calories: 380
Protein: 22 grams
Fat: 26 grams
Carbohydrate: 14 milligrams
Cholesterol: 80 milligrams
Sodium: 95 milligrams
Potassium: 550 milligrams

Food Group Units:
Vegetables: 2
Meat and Alternatives:
      Moderately Low-Fat: 3
Milk Products:
      Moderately Low-Fat: ¼
Fat:
      Monounsaturated: 1
      Saturated: 1

Beef Chop Suey

1 tablespoon vegetable oil
1 pound beef flank steak, cut
   into thin strips

1½ cups diagonally sliced
   celery (3 large stalks)
2 cups red pepper strips
   (1 large red pepper)
½ cup chopped onion
2 garlic cloves, minced
½ teaspoon chopped ginger
   root
1½ cups low-sodium chicken
   broth
1 tablespoon cornstarch
1 tablespoon low-sodium soy
   sauce
¼ teaspoon sugar
⅛ teaspoon pepper
½ cup fresh bean sprouts
2 cups cooked rice

In large non-stick skillet over medium-high heat in hot oil, cook beef about 5 minutes or until browned, stirring frequently; remove from skillet. Add celery, red pepper, onion, garlic, and ginger root to drippings in skillet; cook about 5 minutes or until tender-crisp, stirring occasionally.

In small bowl, combine remaining ingredients, except sprouts and rice; add to skillet. Cook until thickened, stirring occasionally. Add sprouts; cook about 1 minute, stirring frequently. Serve over rice. Makes 4 servings, about 1¼ cups each.

Approximate Nutrient Analysis Per Serving:
Calories: 370
Protein: 29 grams
Fat: 11 grams
Carbohydrate: 37 grams
Cholesterol: 75 milligrams
Sodium: 485 milligrams
Potassium: 790 milligrams

Food Group Units:
Vegetables: 2
Grains: 1½
Meat and Alternatives:
    Moderately Low-Fat: 3

Sauerbraten Stew

1½ pounds beef stew meat
1 cup red wine vinegar
½ cup sliced onions
water
¼ cup dry red wine
1 bay leaf
2 whole cloves
½ teaspoon peppercorns
½ teaspoon salt
1 tablespoon vegetable oil
2 tablespoons all-purpose
  flour
6 gingersnaps, crushed
½ teaspoon sugar
3 cups cooked noodles
  (6 ounces raw)

In shallow dish, place beef.

In medium bowl, combine vinegar, onion, ½ cup water, wine, bay leaf, cloves, peppercorns, and salt; pour over beef and stir well. Cover and refrigerate about 8 hours, stirring occasionally.

Remove beef from marinade, reserving marinade. Dry beef with paper towels. In large saucepan over medium-high heat in hot oil, brown beef. Drain and discard excess fat. Add reserved marinade to saucepan; bring to a boil. Reduce heat; cover. Simmer about 1½–2 hours until beef is tender, stirring occasionally. With slotted spoon, remove beef. Strain liquid. Return liquid to saucepan with beef.

In small bowl, combine flour and ¼ cup water. Add to saucepan; cook about 2–3 minutes or until thickened. Stir in gingersnap crumbs and sugar. Serve over noodles. Makes 6 servings.

Approximate Nutrient Analysis Per Serving:
Calories: 435
Protein: 24 grams
Fat: 23 grams
Carbohydrate: 32 grams
Cholesterol: 100 milligrams
Sodium: 265 milligrams
Potassium: 290 milligrams

Food Group Units:
Grains: 2
Meat and Alternatives:
    Moderately Low-Fat: 3
Fat:
    Polyunsaturated: ½

Caraway Pork Chops

4 loin rib pork chops, cut
    ¾-inch thick
2 small potatoes, peeled and
    chopped (about 10 or 12
    ounces)
½ cup chopped onion
1 16-ounce can tomatoes in
    juice, chopped
½ teaspoon caraway seed
⅛ teaspoon salt
⅛ teaspoon pepper

In large non-stick skillet sprayed with non-stick cooking spray over medium-high heat, brown pork chops. Remove from skillet. Add potatoes and onion to drippings in skillet; cook about 5 minutes, stirring occasionally. Return pork chops to skillet and add remaining ingredients; bring to a boil. Reduce heat; cover. Simmer about 45 minutes to 1 hour or until pork is tender. Transfer pork chops and vegetables to serving platter. Increase heat to high. Cook sauce until reduced slightly and thickened. Serve with pork. Makes 4 servings.

Approximate Nutrient Analysis Per Serving:
Calories: 450
Protein: 24 grams
Fat: 30 grams
Carbohydrate: 20 grams
Cholesterol: 75 milligrams
Sodium: 290 milligrams
Potassium: 925 milligrams

Food Group Units:
Vegetables: 2
Grains: ½
Meat and Alternatives:
    Moderately Low-Fat: 3
Fat:
    Polyunsaturated: 2

Pork and Apples

2 teaspoons vegetable oil
1 pound boneless pork
    shoulder, cut into ¾-inch
    cubes
½ cup sliced onion
1½ cups low-sodium beef
    broth
½ cup unsweetened apple
    juice
1 bay leaf
¼ teaspoon thyme
¼ teaspoon salt
⅛ teaspoon pepper
2 cups sliced celery
2 small apples, peeled, cored
    and sliced
1 tablespoon all-purpose flour
2 tablespoons water

In medium skillet over medium-high heat in hot oil, brown pork. Remove from saucepan. Add onion to drippings in saucepan, cook about 3 minutes or until soft, stirring occasionally. Return pork to saucepan. Add beef broth, apple juice, bay leaf, thyme, salt, and pepper; bring to a boil. Reduce heat; cover. Simmer about 1½ hours, stirring occasionally. Add celery; continue to simmer about 30 minutes or until pork and celery are tender. Add apples; cook about 5 minutes.

In small bowl, combine flour and water. Add to saucepan; cook about 2 minutes or until thickened, stirring frequently. Remove and discard bay leaf. Makes 4 servings.

Approximate Nutrient Analysis Per Serving:
Calories: 420
Protein: 19 grams
Fat: 31 grams
Carbohydrate: 18 grams
Cholesterol: 70 milligrams
Sodium: 275 milligrams
Potassium: 645 milligrams

Food Group Units:
Vegetables: 1
Fruit: 1
Meat and Alternatives:
    Moderately Low-Fat: 3
Fat:
    Polyunsaturated: 1
    Saturated: 1

Vegetables

Sautéed Broccoli

4 teaspoons olive oil
2 large garlic cloves, coarsely
   chopped
4 cups fresh or frozen thawed
   broccoli flowerets
   (2 pounds untrimmed or 2
   10-ounce packages)
⅓ cup low-sodium chicken
   broth
1 tablespoon fresh lemon
   juice
¼ teaspoon grated lemon
   peel
⅛ teaspoon pepper

In large skillet over medium-high heat in hot oil, cook garlic about 30 seconds, stirring constantly. Add broccoli; cook about 1 minute, stirring occasionally.

Add remaining ingredients. Reduce heat; cover. Simmer about 5–7 minutes or until broccoli is tender-crisp. Makes 4 servings, about ⅔ cup each.

Approximate Nutrient Analysis Per Serving:
Calories: 90
Carbohydrate: 9 grams
Protein: 5 grams
Fat: 5 grams
Cholesterol: 0
Sodium: 30 milligrams
Potassium: 375 milligrams

Food Group Units:
Vegetables: 2
Fat:
    Polyunsaturated: 1

Sesame Green Beans

2 teaspoons vegetable oil
1 teaspoon sesame oil
¼ cup thinly sliced scallions
1 garlic clove, minced
1 9-ounce package frozen
   French-style green beans,
   thawed and well drained
   (1½ cups fresh)
¼ teaspoon ground ginger
⅛ teaspoon pepper
⅔ cup fresh bean sprouts
1 tablespoon toasted sesame
   seeds
¼ teaspoon soy sauce

In large skillet over medium-high heat in hot vegetable and sesame oil, cook onion and garlic about 3 minutes or until soft, stirring frequently. Add beans, ginger and pepper; cook about 5 minutes, stirring frequently. Stir in bean sprouts, sesame seeds and soy sauce; cook about 1 minute or until heated through. Makes 4 servings, about ½ cup each.

Approximate Nutrient Analysis Per Serving:
Calories: 70
Protein: 2 grams
Fat: 5 grams
Carbohydrate: 6 grams
Cholesterol: 0
Sodium: 30 milligrams
Potassium: 170 milligrams

Food Group Units:
Vegetables: 1
Fat:
   Monounsaturated: 1

Barbecued Potatoes

1 pound unpeeled potatoes,
   washed (about 2 large)
4 teaspoons margarine,
   melted
1 tablespoon honey
2 teaspoons chili powder
¼ teaspoon garlic powder
⅛ teaspoon pepper

Preheat oven to 425°F.
With a knife, cut potatoes crosswise into thin slices. Place on baking pan sprayed with non-stick cooking spray.
In small bowl, combine remaining ingredients until well blended; spread evenly over potatoes. Bake about 15–20 minutes or until potatoes are fork-tender. Makes 4 servings.

Approximate Nutrient Analysis Per Serving:
Calories: 140
Protein: 3 grams
Fat: 4 grams
Carbohydrate: 25 grams

Cholesterol: 0
Sodium: 60 milligrams
Potassium: 495 milligrams

Food Group Units:
Grains: 1½
Fat:
    Polyunsaturated: 1

Brussels Sprouts with Cream Sauce

2 cups frozen Brussels sprouts
1 tablespoon margarine
1 tablespoon chopped onion
1 garlic clove, minced
1 tablespoon all-purpose flour
½ cup skim milk
1 teaspoon dry white wine
⅛ teaspoon pepper
1½ tablespoons grated
    Parmesan cheese

Cook Brussels sprouts as label directs, omitting salt.
Meanwhile, in small saucepan over low heat, or in double boiler, melt margarine. Add onion and garlic; cook about 3 minutes or until soft, stirring frequently. Add flour; cook about 1 minute, stirring frequently. Gradually add milk, wine, and pepper; cook until thickened and smooth, stirring constantly. Remove from heat; stir in cheese until melted. If sauce becomes too thick, add additional 1–2 tablespoons skim milk. Drain Brussels sprouts; pour sauce over sprouts. Makes 4 servings.

Approximate Nutrient Analysis Per Serving:
Calories: 70
Protein: 4 grams
Fat: 4 grams.
Carbohydrate: 7 grams
Cholesterol: 2 milligrams
Sodium: 90 milligrams
Potassium: 225 milligrams

Food Group Units:
Vegetables: 1½
Fat:
    Polyunsaturated: 1

Sautéed Mixed Vegetables

1 tablespoon margarine
1 teaspoon vegetable oil
1 cup sliced zucchini
    (1 medium)
1 cup red pepper strips
    (½ large)
½ cup sliced celery
    (2–3 small stalks)
¼ cup chopped onion
2 garlic cloves, minced
½ pound mushrooms,
    quartered (3 cups)
¾ teaspoon oregano, crushed
½ teaspoon basil, crushed
⅛ teaspoon salt
⅛ teaspoon crushed red
    pepper (optional)

In large non-stick skillet over medium-high heat, heat margarine and oil. Add zucchini, red pepper, celery, onion, and garlic; cook about 10 minutes or until tender-crisp, stirring frequently. Add remaining ingredients; cook about 3 minutes, stirring constantly. Makes 4 servings, about ¾ cup each.

Approximate Nutrient Analysis Per Serving:
Calories: 80
Protein: 3 grams
Fat: 4 grams
Carbohydrate: 9 grams
Cholesterol: 0
Sodium: 135 milligrams
Potassium: 470 milligrams

Food Group Units:
Vegetables: 2
Fat:
Polyunsaturated: ½

Red Cabbage and Apples

1 tablespoon margarine
¼ cup chopped onion
½ cup water
1 tablespoon white vinegar
¾ teaspoon caraway seeds
½ teaspoon sugar
⅛ teaspoon salt
⅛ teaspoon pepper
2 cups shredded red cabbage
1 small apple, cored and
    sliced

In medium saucepan over medium-high heat, melt margarine. Add onion; cook about 3 minutes or until soft, stirring frequently. Add remaining ingredients; cover. Simmer about 5–7 minutes or until cabbage is tender-crisp, stirring occasionally. Makes 3–4 servings, about ½–1 cup each.

Approximate Nutrient Analysis Per Serving:
Calories: 60
Protein: 1 gram
Fat: 3 grams
Carbohydrate: 8 grams
Cholesterol: 0
Sodium: 115 milligrams
Potassium: 150 milligrams

Food Group Units:
Vegetables: ½
Fruit: ½
Fat:
Polyunsaturated: ½

Snowpeas and Water Chestnuts

4 teaspoons vegetable oil
2 garlic cloves, minced
½ teaspoon finely chopped
    ginger root
1 6-ounce package frozen
    snowpeas, thawed and well
    drained (1½ cups fresh)
⅓ cup sliced water chestnuts
½ cup coarsely chopped red
    pepper
1 teaspoon soy sauce
⅛ teaspoon pepper

In large non-stick skillet over medium-high heat in hot oil, cook garlic and ginger root about 1 minute. Add remaining ingredients; cook about 5–7 minutes or until tender-crisp, stirring frequently. Makes 4 servings, about ½ cup each.

Approximate Nutrient Analysis Per Serving:
Calories: 80
Protein: 2 grams
Fat: 5 grams
Carbohydrate: 9 grams
Cholesterol: 0
Sodium: 115 milligrams
Potassium: 170 milligrams

Food Group Units:
Vegetables: 2
Fat:
    Polyunsaturated: 1

Leeks au Gratin

6 medium leeks, trimmed, cut
    into ¾-inch slices and
    washed
1 tablespoon margarine

133

2 tablespoons all-purpose
  flour
¾ cup skim milk
1 teaspoon dry mustard
⅛ teaspoon pepper
2 tablespoons grated
  Parmesan cheese
1 ounce shredded part-skim
  mozzarella cheese (¼ cup)

Preheat oven to 375°F.

In large skillet over medium heat in 1 inch boiling water, place leek slices in a single layer; heat to boiling. Reduce heat; cover. Simmer about 10 minutes or until tender-crisp; drain. (Do in batches, if necessary.)

In 1½-quart shallow baking dish sprayed with non-stick cooking spray, place leeks.

Meanwhile, in small saucepan over low heat or in double boiler, melt margarine. Add flour; cook about 1 minute, stirring constantly. Gradually add milk, mustard, and pepper; cook until thickened and smooth, stirring constantly.

Remove from heat; stir in Parmesan cheese. Pour over leeks. Sprinkle with mozzarella cheese. Bake about 30 minutes or until hot and bubbly. Makes 6 servings.

Calories: 85
Protein: 4 grams
Fat: 3 grams
Carbohydrate: 9 grams
Cholesterol: 5 milligrams
Sodium: 95 milligrams
Potassium: 235 milligrams

Food Group Units:
Vegetables: 1
Milk Products:
    Very Low-Fat: ½
Fat:
    Polyunsaturated: ½

134

Creamed Mushrooms

2 tablespoons margarine
⅓ cup chopped onion
1 garlic clove, minced
1 pound mushrooms, halved
   (6 cups)
¼ teaspoon rosemary,
   crushed
⅛ teaspoon salt
⅛ teaspoon pepper
2 tablespoons dry white wine
½ cup skim milk
2 teaspoons arrowroot

In large skillet over medium-high heat, melt margarine. Add onion and garlic; cook about 3 minutes or until soft, stirring frequently. Add mushrooms, rosemary, salt, and pepper. Cook about 15 minutes or until liquid has evaporated, stirring occasionally. Add wine; continue to cook until liquid has evaporated, stirring frequently.

In small bowl, combine milk and cornstarch; mix well. Add to skillet; cook about 2–3 minutes or until thickened, stirring constantly. Makes 6 servings, about ⅓ cup each.

Approximate Nutrient Analysis Per Serving:
Calories: 70
Protein: 3 grams
Fat: 4 grams
Carbohydrate: 6 grams
Cholesterol: 0
Sodium: 115 milligrams
Potassium: 370 milligrams

Food Group Units:
Vegetables: 1
Fat:
      Polyunsaturated: 1

Scalloped Tomatoes

1 16-ounce can tomatoes in
  juice, chopped
2 tablespoons minced green
  pepper
2 tablespoons minced onion
1 garlic clove, minced
1 teaspoon basil, crushed
⅛ teaspoon pepper
2 slices stale or day-old whole
  wheat bread, cut into cubes
  (1½ cups)
4 teaspoons margarine,
  melted

Preheat oven to 375°F.

In a 1-quart casserole sprayed with non-stick cooking spray, place tomatoes in juice. Stir in green pepper, onion, garlic, basil, and pepper. In a small bowl, combine bread cubes and margarine; sprinkle over tomatoes. Bake about 30 minutes until hot and bubbly. Makes 4 servings.

Approximate Nutrient Analysis Per Serving:
Calories: 90
Protein: 3 grams
Fat: 4 grams
Carbohydrate: 12 grams
Cholesterol: 0
Sodium: 255 milligrams
Potassium: 315 milligrams

Food Group Units:
Vegetables: 2
Fat:
    Polyunsaturated: 1

Mashed Turnips and Potatoes

3 small potatoes, peeled and
  cubed (12 ounces)
1½ cups peeled, cubed

turnips (about 8 ounces
  unpared)
1–2 tablespoons skim milk
2 tablespoons margarine
1 tablespoon chopped fresh
  parsley
1 tablespoon chopped chives
¼ teaspoon salt
Dash ground red pepper
2 tablespoons grated
  Parmesan cheese

In large saucepan over medium heat in boiling water, cook potatoes and turnips about 20–30 minutes or until fork-tender; drain.

In large bowl, combine potatoes, turnips, milk, and margarine; mash until fluffy. Stir in parsley, chives, salt, and red pepper. Spoon potato mixture into 1-quart shallow baking dish. Sprinkle with cheese. Broil about 3 to 4 inches from heat about 1–2 minutes or until lightly browned. Makes 4 servings, about ½ cup each.

Approximate Nutrient Analysis Per Serving:
Calories: 145
Protein: 4 grams
Fat: 7 grams
Carbohydrate: 18 grams
Cholesterol: 2 milligrams
Sodium: 28 milligrams
Potassium: 505 milligrams

Food Group Units:
Vegetables: 1
Grains: 1
Fat:
    Polyunsaturated: 1

Carrot Soufflé

1 cup chopped carrots (about
  2 carrots)
1 tablespoon margarine

1½ tablespoons all-purpose
  flour
½ cup skim milk
1 teaspoon honey
¼ teaspoon salt
½ teaspoon grated orange
  peel
¼ teaspoon ground cinnamon
⅛ teaspoon pepper
Dash ground nutmeg
2 eggs, separated

In medium saucepan in 1-inch boiling water, heat carrots to boiling. Reduce heat; cover. Simmer about 15 minutes or until tender; drain.

In covered blender or food processor, purée carrots; set aside.

In small saucepan over low heat, or in double boiler, melt margarine. Add flour; cook about 1 minute, stirring constantly. Gradually add skim milk, honey, salt, orange peel, cinnamon, pepper, and nutmeg; cook until thickened and smooth, stirring constantly.

Meanwhile, preheat oven to 325°F.

In a small bowl, beat egg yolks. Beat a small amount of hot mixture into egg yolks; add to saucepan. Cook until thickened, stirring constantly. Stir in purée.

In large bowl, beat egg whites until stiff peaks form; gently fold into carrot mixture. Into 1-quart soufflé dish sprayed with non-stick cooking spray, spoon mixture. Bake about 45–55 minutes or until puffed and lightly browned. Serve immediately. Makes 6 servings.

Approximate Nutrient Analysis Per Serving:
Calories: 70
Protein: 3 grams
Fat: 4 grams
Carbohydrate: 6 grams
Cholesterol: 92 milligrams
Sodium: 155 milligrams
Potassium: 125 milligrams

Food Group Units:
Vegetables: 1

Meat and Alternatives:
    Moderately Low-Fat: ½

Mushroom Strudel

5 tablespoons margarine,
    divided
½ cup chopped onion
1 garlic clove, minced
1½ pounds mushrooms,
    chopped (about 6 cups)
½ teaspoon thyme, crushed
¼ teaspoon salt
⅛ teaspoon pepper
2 tablespoons dry white wine
½ cup plain dry bread crumbs
1 egg white, slightly beaten
12 sheets phyllo leaves

In large non-stick skillet over medium-high heat in 1 tablespoon hot margarine, cook onion and garlic about 3 minutes, stirring occasionally. Add mushrooms, thyme, salt, and pepper; cook about 20 minutes, stirring frequently. Add wine; cook about 5 minutes or until all liquid has evaporated, stirring frequently. Cool to room temperature; stir in bread crumbs and egg white.

Preheat oven to 375°F.

In small saucepan, melt remaining margarine. On damp towel, place one phyllo sheet; brush lightly with margarine. Layer remaining phyllo sheets on top, brushing every other layer with margarine. Spoon mushroom mixture over dough, leaving 2-inch border on all sides. Fold shorter sides toward center. Starting from longer end, roll up. On baking sheet sprayed with non-stick cooking spray, place mushroom strudel seam-side-down; brush with remaining margarine. Bake about 20–30 minutes until golden brown. Cool about 10 minutes on wire rack before slicing. Makes 8 servings.

Approximate Nutrient Analysis Per Serving:
Calories: 230

Protein: 7 grams
Fat: 8 grams
Carbohydrate: 33 grams
Cholesterol: 0
Sodium: 220 milligrams
Potassium: 395 milligrams

Food Group Units:
Vegetables: 2
Grains: 1½
Fat:
    Polyunsaturated: 1½

Salads

Mixed Vegetable Salad

2 cups broccoli flowerets
    (1 pound untrimmed)
½ pound mushrooms, sliced
    (3 cups)
1 cup green pepper strips
    (1 medium)
1 cup red pepper strips
    (1 medium)
¼ cup chopped red onion
¼ cup vegetable oil
2 tablespoons red wine
    vinegar
1 garlic clove, minced
¾ teaspoon basil, crushed
¼ teaspoon thyme, crushed
⅛ teaspoon pepper

In medium saucepan in 1-inch boiling water, heat broccoli to boiling. Reduce heat; cover. Simmer about 3 minutes or until tender-crisp; drain. Rinse under cold running water.

Transfer to large bowl. Add mushrooms, green and red pepper, and onion; toss.

In small bowl, combine oil, vinegar, garlic, basil, thyme, and pepper; pour over vegetables. Toss well. Cover and refrigerate about 2 hours. Makes 6 servings, about 1 cup each.

Approximate Nutrient Analysis Per Serving:
Calories: 120
Protein: 3 grams
Fat: 9 grams
Carbohydrate: 7 grams
Cholesterol: 0
Sodium: 20 milligrams
Potassium: 355 milligrams

Food Group Units:
Vegetables: 1
Fat:
    Polyunsaturated: 2

Cucumber Salad

2 cups peeled and sliced
  cucumbers (1 large)
2 tablespoons minced red
  pepper
2 tablespoons finely chopped
  green onion
3 tablespoons vegetable oil
1 tablespoon white vinegar
1 garlic clove, minced
½ teaspoon dill weed
½ teaspoon sugar
¼ teaspoon salt
⅛ teaspoon pepper

In medium bowl, combine cucumbers, red pepper, and green onion; toss.

In small bowl, combine remaining ingredients; pour over vegetables. Toss well. Cover and refrigerate about 2 hours. Makes 4 servings, about ½ cup each.

Approximate Nutrient Analysis Per Serving:
Calories: 110
Protein: 1 gram
Fat: 11 grams
Carbohydrate: 4 grams
Cholesterol: 0
Sodium: 140 milligrams
Potassium: 140 milligrams

Food Group Units:
Vegetables: 1
Fat:
    Polyunsaturated: 2

Indian Rice Salad

⅔ cup brown rice
½ cup raisins
10 whole almonds, coarsely
    chopped and toasted
¼ cup chopped celery
2 tablespoons chopped onion
3 tablespoons vegetable oil
1½ tablespoons white vinegar
1 garlic clove, minced
1 teaspoon curry powder
½ teaspoon ground cumin
¼ teaspoon ground cinnamon
¼ teaspoon salt
⅛ teaspoon pepper

Cook rice as label directs, omitting salt.

In medium bowl, combine rice, raisins, almonds, celery, and onion; toss.

In small bowl, combine remaining ingredients; pour over salad. Toss well. Cover and refrigerate about 2 hours. Makes 4 servings, about ¾ cup each.

Approximate Nutrient Analysis Per Serving:
Calories: 280
Protein: 4 grams
Fat: 13 grams

Carbohydrate: 40 grams
Cholesterol: 0
Sodium: 150 milligrams
Potassium: 270 milligrams

Food Group Units:
Fruit: 1
Grains: 2
Fat:
    Polyunsaturated: 2½

Creamy Chicken Salad

2 cups chopped cooked
    chicken (1 pound 10 ounces
    raw, trimmed)
¾ cup 1-inch julienne
    zucchini strips (1 small)
½ cup torn spinach leaves
¼ cup chopped carrot
    (1 small)
6 walnut halves, chopped
    (2½ tablespoons)
¼ cup plain low-fat yogurt
2 tablespoons mayonnaise
1 small garlic clove, minced
¼ teaspoon tarragon, crushed
⅛ teaspoon salt
⅛ teaspoon pepper
whole spinach leaves

In medium bowl, combine chicken, zucchini, spinach, carrots, and walnuts; toss.

In small bowl, combine remaining ingredients; pour over salad. Toss well. Cover and refrigerate about 2 hours. Serve on whole spinach leaves. Makes 4 servings, about ¾ cup each.

Approximate Nutrient Analysis Per Serving:
Calories: 225
Protein: 23 grams
Fat: 13 grams

Carbohydrate: 4 grams
Cholesterol: 70 milligrams
Sodium: 190 milligrams
Potassium: 335 milligrams

Food Group Units:
Vegetables: ½
Meat and Alternatives:
    Very Low-Fat: 3
Fat:
    Polyunsaturated: 2

Tofu Salad

¼ cup vegetable oil
2 tablespoons red wine
    vinegar
1 garlic clove, minced
½ teaspoon oregano, crushed
¼ teaspoon salt
⅛ teaspoon crushed red
    pepper
8 ounces tofu (bean curd),
    drained and cut into ½-inch
    cubes (3½ cups)
2 cups chopped tomatoes
    (about 2½ medium
    tomatoes)
¼ pound mushrooms, sliced
    (2 cups)
¼ cup sliced celery (1 large
    stalk)
¼ cup chopped green pepper
¼ cup chopped fresh parsley
2 tablespoons chopped onion

In large bowl, combine oil, vinegar, garlic, oregano, salt, and red pepper; mix well. Add tofu; toss. Cover and refrigerate about 2 hours, stirring occasionally.

About 1 hour prior to serving, add vegetables; toss to coat. Makes 6 servings, about ⅓ cup each.

Approximate Nutrient Analysis Per Serving:
Calories: 135
Protein: 5 grams
Fat: 11 grams
Carbohydrate: 6 grams
Cholesterol: 0
Sodium: 105 milligrams
Potassium: 320 milligrams

Food Group Units:
Vegetables: 1
Meat and Alternatives:
    Moderately Low-Fat: 1
Fat:
    Polyunsaturated: 1

Pasta and Vegetable Salad

4 ounces small shell macaroni
   (1¼ cups dry)
½ cup chopped broccoli
½ cup chopped carrot
¼ cup chopped red pepper
2 tablespoons chopped onion
¼ cup plain low-fat yogurt
1 tablespoon vegetable oil
2 teaspoons white vinegar
1 garlic clove, minced
1½ teaspoons dry mustard
Dash hot pepper sauce
   (optional)
¼ teaspoon salt
⅛ teaspoon pepper

Cook pasta as label directs, omitting salt.

Meanwhile, in medium saucepan in 1-inch boiling water, add broccoli; heat to boiling. Reduce heat; cover. Simmer about 2 minutes or until tender-crisp; drain. Rinse under cold running water.

In large bowl, combine drained pasta with broccoli, carrot, red pepper, and onion; toss.

In small bowl, combine remaining ingredients; pour over salad. Toss well. Cover and refrigerate about 2 hours. Makes 4 servings, about ¾ cup each.

Approximate Nutrient Analysis Per Serving:
Calories: 170
Protein: 6 grams
Fat: 5 grams
Carbohydrate: 27 grams
Cholesterol: 1 milligram
Sodium: 160 milligrams
Potassium: 230 milligrams

Food Group Units:
Vegetables: 2
Grains: 1
Fat:
    Polyunsaturated: 1

Waldorf Salad

2 small apples, cored and
  chopped (1⅓ cups)
2 small pears, cored and
  chopped (1½ cups)
1 small banana, sliced (½ cup)
½ cup chopped celery
  (2 medium stalks)
¼ cup raisins
12 walnut halves, chopped
  (rounded ⅓ cup)
½ cup plain low-fat yogurt
2 tablespoons mayonnaise
1 teaspoon lemon juice

In medium bowl, combine all ingredients; toss well. Cover and refrigerate about 2 hours. Makes 6 servings, about ¾ cup each.

Approximate Nutrient Analysis Per Serving:
Calories: 145

Protein: 2 grams
Fat: 7 grams
Carbohydrate: 21 grams
Cholesterol: 4 milligrams
Sodium: 55 milligrams
Potassium: 285 milligrams

Food Group Units:
Vegetables: ½
Fruit: 2
Fat:
    Polyunsaturated: 1

Red Potato Salad

1 pound small red potatoes
  (about 8)
1 8-ounce can white kidney
  beans, drained and rinsed
1 cup chopped red pepper
  (1 large)
¾ cup sliced celery
  (3 medium stalks)
¼ cup thinly sliced onion
¼ cup vegetable oil
2 tablespoons red wine
  vinegar
1 garlic clove, minced
¾ teaspoon dill weed
¼ teaspoon salt
⅛ teaspoon pepper

In medium saucepan in 1-inch boiling water, add potatoes; heat to boiling. Reduce heat to low; cover. Simmer 15–20 minutes or until fork-tender; drain. Cool to room temperature.

Cut potatoes into quarters; place in large bowl. Add beans, red pepper, celery, and onion; toss.

In small bowl, combine remaining ingredients; pour over salad. Toss well. Cover and refrigerate about 2 hours. Makes 6 servings, about ¾–1 cup each.

Approximate Nutrient Analysis Per Serving:
Calories: 190
Protein: 5 grams
Fat: 10 grams
Carbohydrate: 23 grams
Cholesterol: 0
Sodium: 115 milligrams
Potassium: 535 milligrams

Food Group Units:
Grains: 1
Fat:
    Polyunsaturated: 1½

Confetti Slaw

1½ cups shredded green
    cabbage
½ cup shredded red cabbage
½ cup shredded carrot
2 tablespoons minced onion
2 tablespoons plain low-fat
    yogurt
2 tablespoons mayonnaise
1½ teaspoons skim milk
1½ teaspoons fresh lemon
    juice
¼ teaspoon celery seed
¼ teaspoon salt
¼ teaspoon sugar
⅛ teaspoon pepper

In large bowl, combine green and red cabbage, carrot, and onion; toss.

In small bowl, combine remaining ingredients; pour over salad. Toss well. Cover and refrigerate about 2 hours. Makes 4 servings, about ¾ cup each.

Approximate Nutrient Analysis Per Serving:
Calories: 80
Protein: 1 gram
Fat: 6 grams

Carbohydrate: 6 grams
Cholesterol: 5 milligrams
Sodium: 195 milligrams
Potassium: 185 milligrams

Food Group Units:
Vegetables: 1
Fat:
    Polyunsaturated: 1

Orzo Salad

6 ounces orzo macaroni*
    (1 cup dry)
¾ cup chopped zucchini
    (1 small)
½ cup thinly sliced carrot
    (1 medium)
½ cup sliced celery
    (2 medium stalks)
2 tablespoons chopped onion
¼ cup chopped fresh parsley
2 tablespoons olive oil
1½ tablespoons red wine
    vinegar
1 tablespoon vegetable oil
1 tablespoon grated Parmesan
    cheese
1 garlic clove, minced
½ teaspoon basil, crushed
¼ teaspoon salt
⅛ teaspoon pepper

Cook pasta as label directs, omitting salt.

Meanwhile, in medium saucepan in 1-inch boiling water, add vegetables; heat to boiling. Reduce heat; cover. Simmer about 3 minutes or until tender-crisp; drain. Rinse under cold running water.

In a large bowl, combine drained pasta, vegetables, and parsley; toss.

In small bowl, combine remaining ingredients; pour over

salad. Toss well. Cover and refrigerate about 2 hours. Makes 6 servings, about ½ cup each.

*Small shells or bows may be substituted for orzo.

Approximate Nutrient Analysis Per Serving:
Calories: 185
Protein: 5 grams
Fat: 8 grams
Carbohydrate: 24 grams
Cholesterol: 1 milligram
Sodium: 125 milligrams
Potassium: 190 milligrams

Food Group Units:
Vegetables: 1
Grains: 1

Sauces and Dressings

Barbecue Sauce

1 8-ounce can tomato sauce
1 tablespoon light brown
   sugar
2 tablespoons white vinegar
2 tablespoons minced onion
1½ tablespoons chili powder
1 garlic clove, minced
1 teaspoon powdered
   mustard

In small saucepan over medium heat, cook all ingredients about 15–20 minutes or until slightly thickened, stirring frequently. May be used as marinade or sauce. Makes 8 servings, about 2 tablespoons each.

Approximate Nutrient Analysis Per Serving:
Calories: 24
Protein: 1 gram
Fat: 0
Carbohydrate: 5 grams
Cholesterol: 0
Sodium: 165 milligrams
Potassium: 150 milligrams

Food Group Units:
Vegetables: 1

Clam Sauce

2 6½-ounce cans minced
  clams
4 teaspoons margarine
2 garlic cloves, minced
¼ cup chopped fresh parsley
1 tablespoon fresh lemon
  juice
¼ teaspoon oregano, crushed
⅛ teaspoon pepper
4 teaspoons grated Parmesan
  cheese

Drain clams, reserving juice.
In small saucepan over medium heat, melt margarine. Add garlic; cook about 1 minute, stirring frequently. Add clam juice, lemon juice, parsley, oregano, and pepper; bring to a boil. Reduce heat; cover. Simmer about 10 minutes. Add clams; cover. Simmer about 5 minutes. Serve over hot pasta and sprinkle with Parmesan cheese. Makes 4 servings, about ⅓ cup each.

Approximate Nutrient Analysis Per Serving:
Calories: 95
Protein: 8 grams
Fat: 5 grams
Carbohydrate: 4 grams
Cholesterol: 30 milligrams

Sodium: 600 milligrams
Potassium: 180 milligrams

Food Group Units:
Vegetables: 1
Meat and Alternatives:
    Very Low-Fat: 1
Fat:
    Polyunsaturated: 1

Mushroom Sauce

2 tablespoons margarine
¼ pound mushrooms,
    quartered
2 tablespoons chopped onion
1 tablespoon all-purpose flour
1 cup low-sodium beef broth
¼ cup chopped fresh parsley
2 tablespoons Madeira wine
¼ teaspoon thyme, crushed
⅛ teaspoon salt
⅛ teaspoon pepper

In medium saucepan over medium-high heat, melt margarine. Add mushrooms and onion; cook about 5 minutes, stirring frequently. Add flour; cook about 1 minute, stirring constantly. Gradually add remaining ingredients; bring to a boil. Cook mixture until slightly thickened or about 3–4 minutes, stirring constantly. May be used as a sauce for meats or vegetables. Makes 10 servings, about 2 tablespoons each.

Approximate Nutrient Analysis Per Serving:
Calories: 30
Protein: 1 gram
Fat: 2 grams
Carbohydrate: 2 grams
Cholesterol: 0
Sodium: 60 milligrams
Potassium: 70 milligrams

Food Group Units:
Vegetables: 1

Catsup

1 tablespoon sugar
1½ tablespoons vinegar
1 6-ounce can tomato paste
2 teaspoons Worcestershire
   sauce
¼ teaspoon garlic powder
⅛ teaspoon pepper

In a small bowl, dissolve sugar in vinegar. Add remaining ingredients, blend well. Cover and refrigerate about 2 hours. Makes 12 servings, about 1 tablespoon each.

Approximate Nutrient Analysis Per Serving:
Calories: 15
Protein: 1 gram
Fat: 0
Carbohydrate: 4 grams
Cholesterol: 0
Sodium: 120 milligrams
Potassium: 125 milligrams

Food Group Units:
Vegetables: ½

Chutney

1 cup peeled, finely chopped
   apples (2 small)
1 cup peeled, chopped pears
   (1½ medium)
½ cup raisins
½ cup firmly packed light
   brown sugar
½ cup cider vinegar
⅓ cup chopped onion

1 garlic clove, minced
¾ teaspoon ground cinnamon
½ teaspoon ground ginger
¼ teaspoon ground allspice
¼ teaspoon pepper

In large saucepan, combine all ingredients; bring to a boil. Reduce heat; simmer about 40 minutes or until thickened, stirring occasionally. Makes 16 servings, about 2 tablespoons each.

Approximate Nutrient Analysis Per Serving:
Calories: 55
Protein: 3 grams
Fat: 1 gram
Carbohydrate: 14 grams
Cholesterol: 0
Sodium: 3 milligrams
Potassium: 95 milligrams

Food Group Units:
Fruit: 1½

Spicy Tomato Dressing

1⅓ cups tomato juice
¼ cup red wine vinegar
2 tablespoons vegetable oil
½ teaspoon oregano, crushed
¼ teaspoon thyme, crushed
⅛ teaspoon hot pepper sauce
⅛ teaspoon garlic powder
⅛ teaspoon ground red
  pepper

In covered jar or shaker, combine all ingredients; chill about 2 hours. Shake well before using. Makes 12 servings, about 2 tablespoons each.

Approximate Nutrient Analysis Per Serving:
Calories: 27

Protein: 0
Fat: 2 grams
Carbohydrate: 1 gram
Cholesterol: 0
Sodium: 55 milligrams
Potassium: 65 milligrams

Food Group Units:
Fat:
    Polyunsaturated: ½

Thousand Island Dressing

1 cup plain low-fat yogurt
3 tablespoons mayonnaise
2 tablespoons chili sauce
1 tablespoon skim milk
1 tablespoon minced onion
1 tablespoon minced green
    pepper
⅛ teaspoon garlic powder
⅛ teaspoon pepper

In small bowl, combine all ingredients; cover. Chill about 2 hours. Stir well before serving. Makes 12 servings, about 2 tablespoons each.

Approximate Nutrient Analysis Per Serving:
Calories: 40
Protein: 1 gram
Fat: 3 grams
Carbohydrate: 2 grams
Cholesterol: 3 milligrams
Sodium: 70 milligrams
Potassium: 60 milligrams

Food Group Units:
Fat:
    Polyunsaturated: 1

Creamy Cucumber Dressing

¾ cup plain low-fat yogurt
⅓ cup peeled, seeded and
  minced cucumber
  (½ medium)
3 tablespoons mayonnaise
1 tablespoon finely chopped
  green onion
1 tablespoon skim milk
1 teaspoon white vinegar
1 garlic clove, minced
⅛ teaspoon pepper

In small bowl, combine all ingredients; mix well. Cover and chill about 2 hours. Stir well before serving. Makes 12 servings, about 2 tablespoons each.

Approximate Nutrient Analysis Per Serving:
Calories: 35
Protein: 1 gram
Fat: 3 grams
Carbohydrate: 1 gram
Cholesterol: 3 milligrams
Sodium: 30 milligrams
Potassium: 45 milligrams

Food Group Units:
Fat:
    Polyunsaturated: 1

Poppy Seed Dressing

¼ cup vegetable oil
2 tablespoons white vinegar
1 tablespoon poppy seeds
1 teaspoon sugar
½ teaspoon tarragon, crushed
⅛ teaspoon ground red
  pepper

In a covered jar or shaker, combine all ingredients; chill about 2 hours. Shake well before using. Serve over fruit or vegetable salads. Makes 12 servings, about 2 teaspoons each.

Approximate Nutrient Analysis Per Serving:
Calories: 45
Protein: 0
Fat: 5 grams
Carbohydrate: 0
Cholesterol: 0
Sodium: 0
Potassium: 8 milligrams

Food Group Units:
Fat:
    Polyunsaturated: 1

Orange Fruit Dressing

1 cup plain low-fat yogurt
2 tablespoons mayonnaise
2 tablespoons orange juice
1 tablespoon honey
¼ teaspoon grated orange
    peel
¼ teaspoon ground cinnamon
⅛ teaspoon ground nutmeg
Dash ground red pepper

In small bowl, combine all ingredients. Cover and chill about 2 hours. Stir well before serving. Makes 10 servings, about 2 tablespoons each.

Approximate Nutrient Analysis Per Serving:
Calories: 45
Protein: 1 gram
Fat: 3 grams
Carbohydrate: 4 grams
Cholesterol: 3 milligrams
Sodium: 30 milligrams
Potassium: 60 milligrams

Food Group Units:
Fat:
    Polyunsaturated: 1

Breads

Herbed Bread Swirl

1 tablespoon margarine,
    melted
2 teaspoons oregano, crushed
1 teaspoon basil, crushed
¼ teaspoon garlic powder
1 pound frozen bread dough,
    thawed
¼ cup chopped fresh parsley
1 egg white
1 tablespoon water

In small bowl, combine margarine, oregano, basil, and garlic powder; set aside.

On lightly floured surface, knead dough about 5 minutes. Roll into 12 x 8–inch rectangle. Brush dough with herb mixture, leaving 1-inch border on all sides. Sprinkle with parsley. Starting with narrow edge, roll dough; seal edges. In 8 x 4–inch loaf pan sprayed with non-stick cooking spray, place seam-side down. Cover with towel; set aside in warm place to rise about 4 hours, or until dough rises ½ inch over top of pan.

Meanwhile, preheat oven to 375°F.

Combine egg white and water; beat slightly. Brush over surface of bread. Bake about 30 minutes or until golden brown. Remove bread from pan; cool on wire rack. Makes 12 servings.

Approximate Nutrient Analysis Per Serving:
Calories: 115
Protein: 3 grams
Fat: 3 grams
Carbohydrate: 18 grams
Cholesterol: 2 milligrams
Sodium: 200 milligrams
Potassium: 55 milligrams

Food Group Units:
Grains: 1
Fat:
    Polyunsaturated: 1

Honey Bran Muffins

1½ cups raw unprocessed
   bran, divided
½ cup boiling water
½ cup all-purpose flour
½ cup whole wheat flour
1½ teaspoons baking soda
⅛ teaspoon salt
1 cup buttermilk
¼ cup honey
2½ tablespoons vegetable oil
1 egg
½ cup raisins (optional)*

Preheat oven to 400°F.

In large bowl, stir together ½ cup bran and water; let stand about 5 minutes.

In small bowl, combine remaining bran with flours, baking soda, and salt.

In another small bowl, combine buttermilk, honey, oil, and egg. Add dry and wet ingredients to wet bran; stir just until moistened. Fold in raisins. In a muffin tin sprayed with non-stick cooking spray, pour batter. Bake about 20 minutes or until toothpick inserted comes out clean. Makes 12 muffins.

*Fresh blueberries (⅔ cup) may be substituted for raisins.

Approximate Nutrient Analysis Per Serving:
Calories: 115
Protein: 4 grams
Fat: 4 grams
Carbohydrate: 19 grams
Cholesterol: 25 milligrams
Sodium: 80 milligrams
Potassium: 140 milligrams

Food Group Units:
Fat:
    Polyunsaturated: 1

Cracked Wheat Bread

⅓ cup skim milk, scalded
⅓ cup molasses
3 tablespoons margarine
1 teaspoon salt
1⅓ cups warm water
  (105–115°F)
1 package active dry yeast
4–4½ cups all-purpose flour
¾ cup whole wheat flour
⅔ cup cracked wheat (bulgur)
1 egg white
1 tablespoon water

In small bowl, combine milk, molasses, margarine, and salt.

In large bowl, sprinkle yeast over warm water; set aside about 5 minutes or until yeast dissolves. With wire whisk, beat in milk mixture. Stir in 3 cups all-purpose flour, whole wheat flour, and cracked wheat until smooth. Mix in enough additional all-purpose flour to make a soft dough.

Onto lightly floured surface, turn dough; knead about 10

minutes or until smooth and elastic, adding more flour. In large greased bowl, place dough, turning to expose greased portion. Cover with towel; set aside in warm place to rise until doubled, or about 1½ hours. Punch down dough. With lightly floured rolling pin, roll dough into 12 x 8-inch rectangle. Starting with narrow edge, roll dough; seal edges. In a 9 x 5-inch pan sprayed with non-stick cooking spray, place seam-side-down. Cover with towel; set aside in warm place to rise until doubled, or about 1 hour.

Meanwhile, preheat oven to 375°F.

Combine egg white and water; beat slightly. Brush over surface of dough. Bake about 50 minutes or until golden brown. Remove from pan and cool on wire rack. Makes 18 servings.

Approximate Nutrient Analysis Per Serving:
Calories: 185
Protein: 5 grams
Fat: 2 grams
Carbohydrate: 36 grams
Cholesterol: 0
Sodium: 150 milligrams
Potassium: 140 milligrams

Food Group Units:
Grains: 2½
Fat:
    Polyunsaturated: ½

Potato Rolls

⅓ cup skim milk, scalded
2 tablespoons sugar
2 tablespoons margarine
½ teaspoon salt
⅛ teaspoon pepper
1 teaspoon active dry yeast
⅓ cup warm water (105–115°F)
½ cup mashed potato (1 small
    potato)
2–2½ cups all-purpose flour

In small bowl, combine milk, sugar, margarine, salt, and pepper; cool to lukewarm.

In large bowl, sprinkle yeast over warm water; set aside about 5 minutes or until yeast dissolves. Stir in 1½ cups flour until smooth. Add enough additional flour to make a soft dough.

Onto a lightly floured surface, turn dough; knead about 10 minutes or until smooth and elastic, adding more flour as needed. In greased bowl, place dough, turning over to expose greased portion. Cover with towel; set aside in warm place to rise about 1 hour, or until doubled.

Punch down dough; divide into 12 pieces. Shape into 2-inch balls. With scissors, cut each ball in half, then into quarters, cutting through almost to bottom of rolls. In muffin pan, sprayed with non-stick cooking spray, place each cut potato roll. Cover with towel; set aside in warm place to rise about 45 minutes, or until doubled.

Meanwhile, preheat oven to 400°F.

Bake rolls about 15–20 minutes, or until golden brown. Makes 6 servings, 2 rolls each.

Approximate Nutrient Analysis Per Serving:
Calories: 245
Protein: 6 grams
Fat: 4 grams
Carbohydrate: 45 grams
Cholesterol: 0
Sodium: 235 milligrams
Potassium: 80 milligrams

Food Group Units:
Vegetables: 1
Grains: 2½
Fat:
    Polyunsaturated: 1

Prune and Nut Bread

2 cups all-purpose flour
1 cup whole wheat flour
⅓ cup sugar
4 teaspoons baking powder

¼ teaspoon salt
1½ cups skim milk
1 egg
3 tablespoons margarine,
    melted
1 teaspoon vanilla extract
36 pitted prunes, chopped
    (3 cups chopped)
30 whole shelled almonds,
    chopped

Preheat oven to 325°F.

In large bowl, combine flours, sugar, baking powder and salt; set aside.

In small bowl, combine milk, egg, margarine, and vanilla extract; with fork, beat slightly. Stir in flour mixture until moistened. Gently fold in prunes and almonds; spoon into 9 x 5–inch loaf pan sprayed with non-stick cooking spray. Bake about 45–60 minutes or until cake tester inserted in center comes out clean. Cook in pan about 10 minutes. Remove from pan; cool on wire rack. Makes 18 servings.

Approximate Nutrient Analysis Per Serving:
Calories: 170
Protein: 4 grams
Fat: 4 grams
Carbohydrate: 31 grams
Cholesterol: 15 milligrams
Sodium: 160 milligrams
Potassium: 215 milligrams

Food Group Units:
Fruit: 1
Grains: 1½
Fat:
    Polyunsaturated: 1

Gingerbread

1 cup all-purpose flour
½ teaspoon baking soda
⅛ teaspoon salt

½ teaspoon ground ginger
¼ teaspoon ground cinnamon
⅛ teaspoon ground cloves
⅛ teaspoon ground allspice
3 tablespoons vegetable
 shortening
2 tablespoons sugar
¼ cup molasses
¼ cup boiling water

Preheat oven to 350°F.

In medium bowl, combine flour, baking soda, salt, and spices; set aside.

In large bowl with electric mixer on medium speed, cream shortening and sugar until light and fluffy; beat in molasses and boiling water. Stir in dry ingredients until moistened. Into 8 x 4–inch loaf pan sprayed with non-stick cooking spray, pour batter. Bake about 30–35 minutes or until cake tester inserted in center comes out clean. Cool in pan on wire rack about 10 minutes. Remove from pan and cool completely on rack. Makes 16 servings.

Approximate Nutrient Analysis Per Serving:
Calories: 70
Protein: 1 gram
Fat: 2 grams
Carbohydrate: 11 grams
Cholesterol: 0
Sodium: 25 milligrams
Potassium: 55 milligrams

Food Group Units:
Grains: ½
Fat:
    Monounsaturated: ½

Desserts

Oatmeal Applesauce Cookies

1 cup all-purpose flour
¼ cup quick cooking oats,
   uncooked
¾ teaspoon baking soda
¼ teaspoon ground cinnamon
Dash ground cloves
2 tablespoons margarine
¼ cup sugar
½ cup unsweetened
   applesauce

Preheat oven to 375°F.

In large bowl, combine flour, oats, baking soda, cinnamon and cloves; set aside.

With mixer at low speed, cream margarine and sugar until light and fluffy; beat in egg and applesauce. Stir in dry ingredients until smooth. Onto baking sheets sprayed with non-stick cooking spray, with a teaspoon, drop cookie batter. Bake about 6–8 minutes or until browned. Cool on wire racks. Makes 8 servings, 3 cookies each.

Approximate Nutrient Analysis Per Serving:
Calories: 125
Protein: 2 grams
Fat: 3 grams
Carbohydrate: 22 grams
Cholesterol: 0
Sodium: 55 milligrams
Potassium: 40 milligrams

Food Group Units:
Grains: 1

Fat:
      Polyunsaturated: ½
Sugars: ½

Mocha Meringues

1 egg white, at room
   temperature
⅛ teaspoon cream of tartar
2 tablespoons sugar
¼ teaspoon vanilla extract
1 tablespoon unsweetened
   cocoa
½ teaspoon instant coffee
   powder

Preheat oven to 250°F.

Line baking sheets with foil.

With mixer at high speed in medium bowl, beat egg white and cream of tartar until soft peaks form; gradually add in sugar and vanilla. Gently fold in cocoa and coffee powder. With a teaspoon, drop meringue onto baking sheets 2 inches apart. Bake about 40 minutes, or until firm. Turn off oven. Let cookies cool in oven 1 hour without opening door. Makes 4 servings, 3 cookies each.

Approximate Nutrient Analysis Per Serving:
Calories: 35
Protein: 1 gram
Fat: 0
Carbohydrate: 7 grams
Cholesterol: 0
Sodium: 10 milligrams
Potassium: 40 milligrams

Food Group Units:
Sugars: ½

Apple Crisp

6 small apples, peeled, cored,
   and sliced (about 1½
   pounds)
2 tablespoons fresh lemon
   juice
¼ teaspoon grated lemon
   peel
½ cup all-purpose flour
2 tablespoons light brown
· sugar
1 teaspoon ground cinnamon
¼ teaspoon ground allspice
4 tablespoons margarine,
   softened

Preheat oven to 350°F.

In 9-inch pie plate sprayed with non-stick cooking spray, arrange apples. Sprinkle with lemon juice and lemon peel.

In small bowl, combine flour, brown sugar, cinnamon, and allspice. Cut in margarine with pastry blender until mixture resembles coarse crumbs. Sprinkle over apples. Bake about 30–40 minutes until lightly browned. Makes 6 servings.

Approximate Nutrient Analysis Per Serving:
Calories: 180
Protein: 1 gram

Fat: 8 grams
Carbohydrate: 28 grams
Cholesterol: 0
Sodium: 90 milligrams
Potassium: 150 milligrams

Food Group Units:
Fruit: 2
Grains: ½
Fat:
    Monounsaturated: 1

Orange Sorbet

2 cups orange juice
2 tablespoons fresh lemon
  juice
2 tablespoons sugar
½ teaspoon grated orange
  peel
1 egg white

In small saucepan over low heat, combine orange juice, lemon juice, sugar and orange peel; cook until sugar dissolves. Pour into large bowl; cool to room temperature.

With mixture at high speed in medium bowl, beat egg white until stiff peaks form; gently fold into orange juice. Into a shallow metal pan, pour mixture. Freeze about 2 hours or until partially frozen.

Into medium bowl, spoon mixture. With electric mixer, beat until smooth. Freeze about 3 hours or until solid. Let stand at room temperature about 10 minutes prior to serving. Makes 4 servings.

Approximate Nutrient Analysis Per Serving:
Calories: 85
Protein: 2 grams
Fat: 0
Carbohydrate: 20 grams
Cholesterol: 0
Sodium: 15 milligrams
Potassium: 260 milligrams

Food Group Units:
Fruit: 1
Meat and Alternatives:
    Very Low-Fat: ¼
Sugars: ½

Baked Bananas

2 small bananas, cut in half
  lengthwise
¼ cup raisins

2 tablespoons margarine,
  melted
1 tablespoon light brown
  sugar
½ teaspoon ground allspice
¼ teaspoon ground cinnamon
Dash ground nutmeg

Preheat oven to 450°F.

In 9-inch pie plate, arrange bananas; sprinkle with raisins.

In small bowl, combine remaining ingredients; pour over bananas. Bake about 10–15 minutes or until hot and bubbly. Makes 4 servings.

Approximate Nutrient Analysis Per Serving:
Calories: 135
Protein: 1 gram
Fat: 6 grams
Carbohydrate: 22 grams
Cholesterol: 0
Sodium: 70 milligrams
Potassium: 265 milligrams

Food Group Units:
Fruit: 2
Fat:
    Polyunsaturated: 1

Cherry Cobbler

1 16-ounce can cherries,
  packed in water
2 tablespoons quick-cooking
  tapioca
2 tablespoons light brown
  sugar
¼ teaspoon ground cinnamon
Dash ground cloves
½ cup all-purpose flour
¾ teaspoon baking powder
⅛ teaspoon salt

2 tablespoons margarine
¼ cup skim milk

Preheat oven to 375°F.

In small saucepan, combine cherries in water, tapioca, brown sugar, cinnamon, and cloves; let sit about 15 minutes. Cook over low heat about 15 minutes or until slightly thickened, stirring occasionally. Into 9-inch pie plate, pour mixture.

In small bowl, combine flour, baking powder, and salt; mix well. With pastry blender, cut in margarine until mixture crumbles; stir in milk. Drop dough in 4 mounds over cherries. Bake about 30 minutes or until lightly browned. Makes 6 servings.

Approximate Nutrient Analysis Per Serving:
Calories: 140
Protein: 2 grams
Fat: 4 grams
Carbohydrate: 25 grams
Cholesterol: 0
Sodium: 150 milligrams
Potassium: 145 milligrams

Food Group Units:
Fruit: 1½
Grains: ½
Fat:
     Polyunsaturated: 1
Sugars: ⅓

Fruit Parfaits

2 medium pears, cored and
   coarsely chopped (1½ cups)
2 medium oranges, peeled,
   sectioned, and cut into
   bite-size pieces (1¾ cups)
1 medium banana, sliced
   (1 cup)
1 cup strawberries, sliced
1½ cups raspberries

¾ cup orange juice
½ teaspoon vanilla extract
2 tablespoons crème de cassis
   (optional)

In large bowl, combine fruits.

In small bowl, combine remaining ingredients; pour over fruits and mix well. Cover and refrigerate about 2 hours, stirring occasionally; spoon into parfait glasses with marinade. Makes 6 servings.

Approximate Nutrient Analysis Per Serving:
Calories: 105
Protein: 2 grams
Fat: 0
Carbohydrate: 26 grams
Cholesterol: 0
Sodium: trace
Potassium: 370 milligrams

Food Group Units:
Fruit: 2

Baked Apples

4 small baking apples, cored
   (about 1½ pounds)
2 tablespoons wheat germ
2 tablespoons raisins
6 walnut halves, chopped
¼ teaspoon ground cinnamon
4 teaspoons orange juice
2 teaspoons margarine,
   melted
1 cup water

Preheat oven to 350°F.

With potato peeler, peel apples, starting from stem end, ⅓ of the way down. In 8-inch square baking dish, arrange apples.

In small bowl, combine wheat germ, raisins, walnuts, and cinnamon. Fill cavities of apples with mixture. Drizzle orange juice and margarine over apples. Pour water in bottom of dish. Bake about 45 minutes or until fork-tender. Makes 4 servings.

Approximate Nutrient Analysis Per Serving:
Calories: 160
Protein: 2 grams
Fat: 5 grams
Carbohydrate: 30 grams
Cholesterol: 0
Sodium: 25 milligrams
Potassium: 270 milligrams

Food Group Units:
Fruit: 2
Grains: ½
Fat:
  Polyunsaturated: 1

Pears with Chocolate Mint Sauce

1½ cups water
½ cup dry white wine
6 small pears, pared and
  cored (about 2¼ pounds)
2 tablespoons unsweetened
  cocoa
2 tablespoons water
1 tablespoon sugar
2½ teaspoons cornstarch
1 cup evaporated skimmed
  milk
⅛ teaspoon mint extract

In large saucepan, heat water and wine to boiling; add pears. Cover; simmer about 30–40 minutes until tender.

Meanwhile, in small saucepan, mix cocoa, water, sugar, and cornstarch; stir in milk. Heat over low heat, until thickened, stirring constantly. Remove from heat; add mint extract. Cover and refrigerate about 2 hours. Transfer pears to serving plate. Serve with sauce. Makes 6 servings.

Approximate Nutrient Analysis Per Serving:
Calories: 145
Protein: 4 grams
Fat: 1 gram
Carbohydrate: 33 grams
Cholesterol: 2 milligrams
Sodium: 5 milligrams
Potassium: 380 milligrams

Food Group Units:
Fruit: 1
Grains: 1½

Strawberry Chiffon Dessert

1½ cups fresh or frozen,
   unsweetened strawberries,
   thawed
1 envelope unflavored gelatin
½ cup cold water
½ cup orange juice
2 tablespoons sugar
1 tablespoon rum
1 teaspoon vanilla extract
2 egg whites

In covered blender or food processor, purée strawberries; set aside.

In small saucepan, sprinkle gelatin over cold water; set aside about 5 minutes or until gelatin softens. Cook over low heat about 5 minutes or until gelatin dissolves, stirring constantly; pour into large bowl. Cool about 5 minutes; beat in orange juice, sugar, rum, vanilla extract, and puréed strawberries. Cover and refrigerate about 1 hour, or until mixture mounds slightly when dropped from a spoon.

In medium bowl with mixer at high speed, beat egg whites until stiff peaks form. Gently fold into gelatin mixture; spoon into parfait glasses. Refrigerate until firm. Makes 4 servings.

Approximate Nutrient Analysis Per Serving:
Calories: 80

Protein: 4 grams
Fat: 0
Carbohydrate: 14 grams
Cholesterol: 0
Sodium: 30 milligrams
Potassium: 175 milligrams

Food Group Units:
Fruit: 1
Meat and Alternatives:
    Very Low-Fat: ½
Sugars: ½

Choco-Banana Cream Puffs

¾ cup water, divided
2 tablespoons margarine
½ cup all-purpose flour
2 eggs
2 teaspoons unflavored
    gelatin
1 small banana, mashed
2 tablespoons unsweetened
    cocoa
2 tablespoons sugar
1 cup plain low-fat yogurt
½ teaspoon vanilla extract
⅛ teaspoon ground cinnamon

Preheat oven to 375°F.

In small saucepan over high heat, cook ½ cup water and margarine to boiling. Reduce heat to low; with wooden spoon, vigorously stir in flour until mixture forms ball and leaves side of pan; remove from heat. Add eggs, one at a time, beating well after each addition until smooth. Onto baking sheet sprayed with non-stick cooking spray, drop batter in 6 large mounds, about 3 inches apart. Bake about 30 minutes or until puffy and golden brown. Cut off tops and reserve. Remove and discard soft dough in center. Cool on wire racks.

Meanwhile, in small saucepan, sprinkle gelatin over remaining ¼ cup cold water; set aside about 5 minutes or until gelatin softens. Cook over low heat about 5 minutes or until gelatin dissolves, stirring constantly; pour into medium bowl, cool 3 minutes. Beat in banana, cocoa, and sugar until smooth. Stir in yogurt, vanilla extract, and cinnamon. Cover and refrigerate. Spoon an equal amount of mixture into cream puffs. Cover with tops. Makes 6 servings.

Approximate Nutrient Analysis Per Serving:
Calories: 160
Protein: 6 grams
Fat: 7 grams
Carbohydrate: 20 grams
Cholesterol: 95 milligrams
Sodium: 95 milligrams
Potassium: 210 milligrams

Food Group Units:
Grains: 1
Meat and Alternatives:
    Very Low-Fat: ½
Fat:
    Polyunsaturated: 1
Sugars: ½

Peach Yogurt Pie

16 2½-inch graham crackers,
  crushed (about 1 cup)
¼ cup bran flakes, crushed
10 teaspoons margarine,
  melted
¼ teaspoon ground cinnamon
1 envelope unflavored gelatin
⅔ cup unsweetened apple
  juice
1 20-ounce package frozen,
  unsweetened peaches,
  thawed and drained (about
  3 cups)
1½ cups plain low-fat yogurt
¼ cup sugar
1 teaspoon vanilla extract
¼ teaspoon ground nutmeg

Preheat oven to 350°F.

In small bowl, combine graham cracker and bran flakes crumbs, margarine, and cinnamon; spoon into 9-inch pie plate, pressing down firmly. Bake about 8–10 minutes or until browned. Cool on wire rack.

In small saucepan, sprinkle gelatin over apple juice; set aside about 5 minutes, or until gelatin softens. Cook over low heat about 5 minutes or until gelatin dissolves, stirring constantly; pour into large bowl.

In covered blender or food processor, purée 2 cups peaches; stir into gelatin. Add with yogurt, sugar, vanilla, and nutmeg; stir until smooth. Cover and refrigerate about 40 minutes or until mixture mounds when dropped from a spoon.

Coarsely chop remaining peaches; fold into gelatin mixture. Spoon into pie crust and refrigerate until firm. Makes 8 servings.

Approximate Nutrient Analysis Per Serving:
Calories: 200
Protein: 5 grams
Fat: 7 grams
Carbohydrate: 31 grams
Cholesterol: 3 milligrams
Sodium: 190 milligrams
Potassium: 330 milligrams

Food Group Units:
Fruit: 1
Grains: 1
Fat:
    Polyunsaturated: 1¼
Sugars: ½

Rice Pudding Mold

2 envelopes unflavored
    gelatin
1 cup cold water, divided
2 cups warm skim milk
¼ cup sugar
2 teaspoons vanilla extract

1 teaspoon ground cinnamon
⅛ teaspoon ground allspice
⅛ teaspoon salt
2 cups cooked rice
½ cup non-fat dry milk

In small saucepan, sprinkle gelatin over ½ cup cold water; set aside about 5 minutes or until gelatin softens. Cook over low heat about 5 minutes or until gelatin dissolves, stirring occasionally. Into a large bowl, pour mixture; cool 5 minutes. Beat in warm milk, sugar, vanilla extract, cinnamon, allspice, and salt; stir in rice. Cover and refrigerate about 50 minutes, or until mixture mounds slightly when dropped from a spoon.

In chilled bowl with chilled beaters, beat non-fat dry milk and remaining cold water until soft peaks form; fold into rice mixture. Into 1½-quart mold sprayed with non-stick cooking spray, spoon mixture. Cover and refrigerate about 8 hours. Invert onto serving plate. Serve with fresh fruit, if desired. Makes 8 servings.

Approximate Nutrient Analysis Per Serving:
Calories: 130
Protein: 6 grams
Fat: 0
Carbohydrate: 24 grams
Cholesterol: 2 milligrams
Sodium: 95 milligrams
Potassium: 200 milligrams

Food Group Units:
Grains: 1½

Pavlova

3 egg whites, at room
   temperature
⅛ teaspoon cream of tartar
⅓ cup sugar
1 teaspoon vanilla extract,
   divided
½ cup nonfat dry milk
½ cup ice water

1½ cups fresh or frozen
   unsweetened strawberries,
   thawed and sliced
1 cup kiwi slices

Preheat oven to 250°F.

Line baking sheet with parchment or brown paper. Draw
an 8-inch circle in center; set aside.

With mixer at high speed, in large bowl beat egg whites and
cream of tartar until soft peaks form; gradually add sugar and
½ teaspoon of vanilla. Spoon meringue in center of circle on
baking sheet; spread to edge of circle, forming 1½-inch rim.
Bake 1¼ hours or until firm. Turn off oven. Let meringue
cool in oven 2 hours without opening door.

In chilled bowl with chilled beaters, beat non-fat dry milk,
water, and remaining vanilla until stiff peaks form; spread
over meringue. Arrange kiwi fruit over top. Makes 8 servings.

Approximate Nutrient Analysis Per Serving:
Calories: 75
Protein: 3 grams
Fat: 0
Carbohydrate: 16 grams
Cholesterol: 1 milligram
Sodium: 45 milligrams
Potassium: 205 milligrams

Food Group Units:
Fruit: 1½
Meat and Alternatives:
     Very Low-Fat: ½
Sugars: ½

Chapter VI

ON YOUR OWN

By reading this book, you have already taken the first steps toward changing diet, behavior, and exercise patterns. These chapters will guide you on the path to living well. But following that path is up to you. Only you have the power to take charge and follow through on your new plan for better health.

Keep in mind the factors that increase risk for atherosclerosis and coronary heart disease in persons who, like you, have been diagnosed as having elevated cholesterol. Cigarette smoking, obesity, insufficient exercise, high blood pressure, and diabetes all compound the danger of disease in a person who also has the major risk factor of high cholesterol. How fortunate that you can eliminate or control these risk factors by simply making the one-day-at-a-time choice to live a healthy life.

Millions of Americans have already made this choice, shifting toward vegetables, fruit, fish, and chicken and away from the saturated fats found in meat, butter, lard, milk, and cream. According to the U.S. Department of Agriculture, there has been a marked improvement in per capita consumption of products affecting CHD risks. Since 1960, use of eggs is down 21 percent, fluid milk and cream down 19 percent, and butter down 43 percent.[5] Consumption of fish and chicken are up 20 percent and 26 percent, respectively.[6,7]

Purchase of low-fat and skim milk products has increased by 300 percent since 1970.[10]

Advice from the Framingham Heart Study, a recent epidemiologic study on heart disease and diet, states: "If Americans would smoke less, get more regular exercise, keep their weight normal, follow a diet lower in fats, and take care of their blood pressure, they would have better chances of avoiding, or at least postponing, heart problems."[4]

Diet alone—monitoring intake of calories, cholesterol, fats, and sodium—can go a long way in lessening the possibility of atherosclerosis and coronary heart disease. For example, overweight and high blood pressure go hand in hand. And in addition to aiding weight control through reducing fluid retention, lowering sodium intake is an important step in lowering blood pressure.

Diabetes, another risk factor, may often be controlled by diet. Just losing weight will bring certain types of diabetes under control.

A healthful diet combined with exercise is doubly effective in helping to guard your health. Studies have shown that exercise alone helps keep cholesterol levels low.

For one study, Finnish lumberjacks consumed about 4,760 calories daily, with a high proportion of their fat obtained from animal sources. Yet their blood cholesterol levels were no higher than those of other men in the same area who ate less fat. The Finnish researchers believe that physical activity was an important factor in keeping cholesterol levels low.[11]

After receiving your doctor's approval, it is recommended that you begin your exercise program with walking. As soon as you get the medical okay, get started! You don't need trendy, expensive clothes; you don't need a team, an opponent, or a partner; you don't need to drive anywhere, invest in equipment, or join costly clubs. All you have to do is step out your front door to start on the path toward living healthfully.

Changing what you eat and increasing your exercise usually requires special effort. In Chapter II, Dr. Foreyt showed you how to change your behavior to make this task easier. With behavior modification, you prepare yourself for dieting and give yourself the tools to stick to your new diet plan.

Just as it helps to talk to friends who are also changing their behavior, it can be beneficial to talk to yourself. Listen to what you are saying to yourself. Are you talking positively, helping yourself make changes in your behavior? Or are you saying negative things that will chip away at your determination and perseverance?

Remind yourself frequently that changing eating habits takes time. Review all the changes you have made so far and pat yourself on the back. Dr. Foreyt's behavior modification method, which rewards good behavior rather than punishing you when you slip up, puts you on the road to correcting ingrained eating habits that may be harmful to your health.

The Beginning

This book has shown you how to guard your heart health by paying attention to two things: diet and exercise. By following a sensible, nutritionally balanced diet, you can control your weight. By establishing a regular exercise program, you can strengthen and tone your body. At the same time, you will burn calories at a more rapid rate, making your weight control task easier. Finally, by following the behavior modification program outlined in this book, you give yourself the tools needed to fit your diet and exercise pattern into your daily life, for better health the rest of your life.

If something is wrong with your car, you fix it. Why not do the same for yourself?

Appendix A

*Cholesterol Content in Foods**

Food Group Units	Low (0–25 mg)	Medium (26–50 mg)	High (50+ mg)
Vegetables	All		
Fruits	All		
Grains	Bread, sandwich	Egg noodles	
	Bread sticks		
	Cereal, dry and hot		
	Graham crackers		
	English muffins		
	Pasta and noodles (non-egg based)		
	Rice		
	Rolls, soft and hard		
Legumes	All		
Meats and Alternatives	Chicken, without skin	Cheese, hard (1 ounce)	Lamb
	Peanut butter	Cottage cheese, creamed	Beef
	Luncheon meats	Chicken, with skin	Pork
	Cheese spreads	Fish, except shrimp	Shrimp
	Cheese food products		Eggs
			Organ meats

183

Milk Products	Evaporated milk, skim or low-fat	
	Skim milk	
	Yogurt, plain (skim and low-fat)	
	Low-fat milk, 1% and 2%	
Fats	Margarine	Butter
	Mayonnaise	Lard
	Salad dressing, except cheese-based	

*Based on commonly eaten portion sizes, with data obtained from *Bowes & Church's Food Values of Portions Commonly Used,* by Jean A. Pennington and Helen Nicholas Church, Philadelphia, J.B. Lippincott Company, 1980.

Appendix B

Types of Fats in Common Fat Products*

High in Polyunsaturates	High in Monounsaturates	High in Saturates	High in Saturates & Cholesterol
• Hollywood safflower oil	• Olive oil	• Crisco hydrogenated shortening	• Butter
• Sunlight safflower oil	• Partially hydrogenated vegetable shortening	• Coconut oil	• Lard
• Soybean oil	• Peanut oil	• Palm oil	• Beef fat
• Mazola corn oil	• Stick margarines, made with partially hydrogenated oil	• Bacon drippings	
• Cottonseed oil	• Imitation margarine	• Meat drippings	
• Tub margarine, made with safflower oil			
• Sesame seed oil			
• Mayonnaise			
• Salad dressing, without cheese			

*Products are listed from highest to lowest content of fat type in each category.

Appendix C

Sodium Content in Foods*

Food Group Units	Low (0–100 mg)	Medium (101–500 mg)	High (500+ mg)
Vegetables	All, except canned and frozen	Canned and frozen	
Fruits	All		
Grains	Cereal, dry Graham crackers Pasta and noodles Rice	Bread sticks Bread, sandwich Rolls, soft and hard Cereal, hot English muffins Muffins Cornbread	
Legumes	All, except canned	Canned	
Meats and Alternatives	Organ meats Eggs Fish, including shellfish Chicken, with and without skin Turkey, with and without skin Beef, except canned, frozen, and dried	Pork Peanut butter Cheese, hard Luncheon meats Cheese food products	Cottage cheese Tuna, packed in oil or water Beef, canned, frozen, and dried

Milk Products		Evaporated milk, skim or low-fat
		Low-fat milk, 1% and 2%
		Skim milk
		Yogurt, plain (skim and low-fat)
Fats	Mayonnaise	Lard
	Margarine	Butter
		Salad dressings

*Based on commonly eaten portion sizes, with data obtained from *Bowes & Church's Food Values of Portions Commonly Used,* by Jean A. Pennington and Helen Nicholas Church, Philadelphia, J.B. Lippincott Company, 1980.

Bibliography

1. American Heart Association: "Risk Factors and Coronary Disease: A Statement for Physicians." *Circulation* 62:445A–451A, 1980.

2. Grande, Francisco, et al.: "Sucrose and Various Carbohydrate-Containing Foods and Serum Lipids in Man." *American Journal of Clinical Nutrition* 27:1043–1051, 1974.

3. Robertson, D.L., et al.: "Epidemiologic Studies of Coronary Heart Disease and Stroke in Japanese Men in Japan, Hawaii and California. Coronary Heart Disease Risk Factors in Japan and Hawaii." *American Journal of Cardiology* 39:244–249, 1977.

4. McDade, Walter: "Good News from the House on Lincoln Street." *Fortune,* pages 86–92, January 14, 1980.

5. United States Department of Agriculture Economic Research Service: "Food Consumption, Prices and Expenditures." *Statistical Bulletin,* pages 127, 671, 672, September 1981.

6. United States Department of Commerce: *Statistical Abstract of the U.S., 1982–1983.* Washington, D.C., U.S. Government Printing Office, page 706, 1983.

7. Commodity Research Bureau, Inc.: *Commodity Year Book, 1983,* page 65, May 1983.

8. General Mills: "A Status Report on the American Diet and Health—1980." Minneapolis, General Mills Nutrition Department, pages 7–8, 1980.

9. Grundy, Scott, et al.: "Rationale of the Diet-Heart Statement of the American Heart Association." *Circulation* 65:839A–854A, 1982.

10. Peterkin, Betty, et al.: "Food Patterns—Where Are We Headed?" *Food from Farm to Table, 1982 Year Book of Agriculture.* Washington, D.C., U.S. Government Printing Office, page 230, 1982.
11. "Diet and Serum Cholesterol Levels of Lumberjacks." *Nutrition Reviews* 20:4–5, 1962.